"*The Pain Reprocessing Therapy Workbook* offers a concise yet powerful approach to reverse chronic neuroplastic pain syndromes. The authors have blended sophisticated neuroscientific principles with a practical approach that will help you recover."

—**Howard Schubiner, MD**, clinical professor at Michigan State University College of Human Medicine, and author of *Unlearn Your Pain*

"Millions of people suffer from real pain or illness in the body that is generated by the brain due to unrecognized life stresses. Fortunately, the new treatment techniques described so clearly in this book by its highly experienced authors can provide relief even for people who have lost hope. Highly recommended."

—**David D. Clarke, MD**, clinical assistant professor of gastroenterology emeritus at Oregon Health & Science University, president of the Psychophysiologic Disorders Association (PPDA), and author of *They Can't Find Anything Wrong!*

"*The Pain Reprocessing Therapy Workbook* is an innovative, comprehensive, and expansive resource for chronic pain relief that strikes a chord across diverse individuals and circumstances. Blackstone and Sinaiko have blended scientifically backed guidance and highly effective exercises with a transformational way of thinking about your pain, yourself, and your relationship to your body. This workbook is an invaluable tool for anyone seeking profound and lasting relief from chronic pain."

—**Christie Uipi, LCSW**, psychotherapist, and founder of The Better Mind Center

"I owe a large part of my recovery from neuroplastic pain to Vanessa's guidance. Early on, she told me, 'There will come a time when you won't even be talking about your pain.' And she was right. Freedom from pain came sooner than I could have imagined. This fantastic workbook will give many more people access to the authors' collective wisdom."

—**Catherine Oxenberg**, mother of three beautiful girls, award-winning actress, and author of *Captive*

"This book is a new and exciting contribution to our understanding of pain reprocessing therapy (PRT). Its practical, easily understandable style will be a huge help for those seeking to learn in a fresh and dynamic way. The writing is engaging and compelling, drawing the reader into a greater depth of knowledge to apply with those who hurt."

—**Martha Teater, LMFT, LCAS, LPC**, licensed behavioral health clinician, author, consultant, and international trainer in the area of chronic pain treatment

"The majority of my patients with chronic pain have neuroplastic pain mechanisms, and will benefit from having this workbook to learn and practice PRT. It's like having a therapist on their side, and there is no one better than Vanessa and Olivia to guide them; they have the practical knowledge and a solid understanding of the neuroscience of pain."

—**Andrea Furlan, MD, PhD**, professor in the department of medicine at the University of Toronto, and author of *8 Steps to Conquer Chronic Pain*

"*The Pain Reprocessing Therapy Workbook* is an essential guide for anyone suffering from chronic pain. The authors have expertly translated the principles of PRT into an easy-to-follow prescription for pain elimination, with many invaluable techniques, tools, and exercises. This workbook will empower those suffering from chronic pain to take control of their pain and symptoms and finally get relief!"

—**Laura Payne, PhD**, assistant professor of psychology at Harvard Medical School, and clinical psychologist and director of the Clinical and Translational Pain Research Lab at McLean Hospital

"This workbook translates the scientifically robust principles of PRT into a user-friendly, step-by-step manual—with heart! People suffering from neural circuit dizziness and other symptoms will find it so practical and reassuring—no screens or tech knowledge required, just willingness to do the work. The principles are thoughtfully supported by practical exercises, and walk the reader through a clear and effective plan for recovery from chronic symptoms."

—**Yonit Arthur, AuD**, audiologist, vestibular specialist, and coach and founder of The Steady Coach

"There have been a lot of advances in our understanding of chronic pain over the previous twenty years. We now realize that taking a pill to reduce pain has been largely ineffective, but reprocessing your central nervous system can reduce your pain and change your life. Vanessa and Olivia's book will lead you through that process and enable you to heal yourself and reclaim your life.

—**Don Teater, MD, MPH**, pain and addiction specialist at Southeast Alaska Regional Health Consortium (SEARHC)

"Neurology is a very young science, and like all new scientific undertakings, practitioners often must invent their personal approach to deal with matters that are still difficult to conceive and describe. This interesting workbook does just that as it creatively asks those who suffer chronic pain to think through how reconceptualizing the neurological basis of their pain might serve to eliminate some significant degree of their suffering."

—**J. W. Freiberg, PhD, JD**, Trauma Research Foundation board member; and author of *Four Seasons of Loneliness, Surrounded by Others and Yet So Alone,* and *Growing Up Lonely*

THE PAIN REPROCESSING THERAPY WORKBOOK

Using the Brain's Neuroplasticity to
Break the Cycle of Chronic Pain

VANESSA M. BLACKSTONE, LCSW

OLIVIA S. SINAIKO, LPC

New Harbinger Publications, Inc.

Publisher's Note

NEW HARBINGER PUBLICATIONS is a registered trademark of New Harbinger Publications, Inc.

New Harbinger Publications is an employee-owned company.

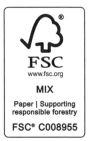

Copyright © 2024 by Vanessa M. Blackstone and Olivia S. Sinaiko
New Harbinger Publications, Inc.
5720 Shattuck Avenue
Oakland, CA 94609
www.newharbinger.com

Cover design by Amy Daniel

Graphics designed by Joshua Wells

Acquired by Wendy Millstine and Ryan Buresh

Edited by Brady Kahn

Printed in the United States of America

26   25   24

10   9   8   7   6   5   4   3   2   1   First Printing

To our grandmothers, the pillars of strength and wisdom whose love and guidance have shaped us into who we are today: Angie, Barbara, Myrna, Norma, and Letes. Some are with us in person, and some in spirit, but all are forever a part of us.

Josh, my anchor, my home, my safety, and the one who teaches me to stand tall. And to Grandpa Harvey "4.0," whose dedication to me ignited a flame to change the world.—V. M. B.

For everyone who has ever cared for me through a migraine, and especially for CKR, whose presence is more soothing than the coldest ice pack.—O. S. S.

Contents

Foreword

In March of 2017, I was at a conference in Michigan, brainstorming with some colleagues about a name for our new treatment. "It needs a name," I said. "Something that captures how the brain can unlearn chronic pain."

After several hours, it was settled. We were going to call it "neuroplastic pain reprocessing therapy." Sure, it was a little wordy, but it conveyed everything we wanted it to.

The next day at the conference, a sporty-looking neuroscientist named Yoni Ashar walked up to me. Yoni would go on to become the lead author of our biggest clinical study to date. "What do you call this treatment?" he asked. "Neuroplastic pain reprocessing therapy," I said, barely able to contain my pride.

Yoni thought for a moment and said, "Drop the 'neuroplastic,' it's cleaner." Then he turned around and walked away.

And I suppose that's the day that pain reprocessing therapy was born.

What is pain reprocessing therapy (PRT)? Well to understand that, you need to know how pain works.

When you sprain your ankle, there are nerve endings in your body that send danger signals to your brain, and pain is generated. This is a good thing. It keeps you from walking on it for a few days, so your ankle can heal.

But sometimes the brain can make a mistake. Sometimes the brain can misinterpret safe signals coming from the body, as if they were dangerous, and generate pain even though the body is fine.

We call this *neuroplastic pain*. And recent studies have found that most forms of chronic pain are, in fact, neuroplastic.

So what does PRT do?

During that same Michigan conference in 2017, I did a live demo with a nurse practitioner named Felicia. Felicia had had chronic neck pain for twenty years. During the live demo, she implemented the techniques of PRT, and her neck pain disappeared!

Yoni came up to me during the break and said, "This is nuts! It's like faith healing but with science."

And it is science.

PRT is a set of techniques that teaches the brain to correctly interpret the signals coming from the body. And that deactivates the pain.

Vanessa M. Blackstone, LCSW, has been treating patients using PRT since the treatment's inception. As the executive director of the Pain Psychology Center, she has helped patients overcome every type of pain imaginable. And now, in partnership with her trusted colleague and collaborator Olivia S. Sinaiko, LPC, she's taken her vast skills and experience and created an excellent PRT workbook to help others recover as well.

There are sixty million chronic pain sufferers in the US, and fifty million of them don't have to be. If you're among them, I implore you to give this book a try. With great skill and clarity, *The Pain Reprocessing Therapy Workbook* lays out the tools and techniques you'll need to overcome your own pain.

—Alan Gordon, LCSW
Founder, Pain Psychology Center

CHAPTER 1

Reprocessing Your Pain

The room is dark. The blackout curtains drawn, the television off, and the phone brightness turned all the way down. There is no noise other than the reassuring voice of the therapist on the other end of the phone. "Clara,"[1] in her first session with the Pain Psychology Center, speaks softly:

> *Where do I begin? Do I describe it as insufferable? Because I'm suffering. I'm still here, but I can't take it anymore. I want to beg and ask to be put out of my misery. At the same time, the idea of giving up almost feels worse. I know it doesn't really make sense, but the light hurts my head so bad that shutting it out almost helps my back feel better. Which helps my feet feel better. How can a change of light calm parts of my body that aren't really a part of why I have pain there? All I know is that I need a solution. I'm not sure why this happened to me, but if I knew, you bet I would have avoided what caused it by all means necessary. I am trying to remember that this won't be forever, but somehow it's really hard to hear that optimistic voice—and I think because the pain is simply so loud. As much as I hate my suffering, knowing that I am not alone has really helped. Because wow, does this feel isolating! I often feel like I am the only person in the world who knows pain like this. Yet, I am angry that I haven't figured out a solution yet.*

Amid the shadows of Clara's journey, we enter the realm of chronic pain.

Chronic pain is indiscriminate, affecting approximately 10 percent of the world's population. Within the United States, an astounding 21 percent of people grapple with chronic pain symptoms that cast a shadow over their daily lives. Symptoms can be described as, but

---

1 All of the clients in this book have given permission for their stories to be presented. Their names have been changed to protect their identities.

not limited to, fatigue, restlessness, dizziness, irritable bowels, aching tendons and muscles, pounding migraines, tension headaches, inflammation, numbness, sharp sensations, dull aches, burning mouth and tongue, and tension or tightness. These symptoms can be consistent over time or ebb and flow in intensity, varying in relationship with different factors like stress, weather, and time of day. As stated by Raffaeli and Arnaudo (2017), the attempt to understand pain represents one of the oldest challenges in the history of medicine.

This workbook, filled with stories, examples, and exercises, is partly a reminder that your journey is shared. You are not alone. And your pain is real. Whether you find yourself at the gym, your local coffee shop, your office, or on the block where you live, consider this: 10 to 20 percent of the people around you also experience chronic pain to some degree.

The prevalence of pain highlights the difficulty of treating a condition that can feel both mysterious and endless. And yet, there is a solution to this seemingly endless cycle of debilitating symptoms. Let's begin by taking a look at the research that proves it.

A Revolutionary Approach

The randomized clinical trial commonly referred to as the "Boulder Back Pain Study," which aimed to treat fifty adults with primary chronic back pain, asked a key question: "Can a psychological treatment based on the reappraisal of primary chronic back pain as due to nondangerous central nervous system processes provide substantial and durable pain relief?" (Ashar et al. 2022). The results showed that two-thirds of participants who received the psychological treatment were pain-free or nearly pain-free afterward, with effects maintained at a one-year follow-up. Images of participants' brains revealed reduced responses to back pain in specific brain regions as well as increased connectivity associated with pain reappraisal. In other words, the study answered its question with a resounding yes: changing the way that people think about their pain can lead to substantial and enduring pain relief.

What was this psychological treatment that so profoundly changed the way people experienced pain? It is an approach that has changed both of our lives, in so many ways. Developed by therapist Alan Gordon, pain reprocessing therapy (PRT) is a therapeutic intervention designed to alleviate chronic pain by challenging patients' beliefs about its causes. The primary goal of PRT is to help chronic pain sufferers recognize that their chronic pain is actually a false alarm that originates in the brain, and not in structural damage in the body. This is a system of techniques, rooted in neuroscience, focused on "embracing a new perspective", as Gordon states in his book *The Way Out*. You will hear more in the next chapter about how exactly pain works. For now, we will begin to understand what this modality is all about.

Contrary to traditional beliefs that chronic pain is solely rooted in structural issues in the body, contemporary studies emphasize the role of psychophysiologic processes in conditions such as chronic back pain, neck pain, fibromyalgia, repetitive strain injury, headaches, TMJ, irritable bowel syndrome, and many others. This paradigm shift recognizes that pain is not always an accurate indicator of ongoing tissue or structural damage but can be a result of the brain misinterpreting harmless signals as threats.

Building on these insights, PRT harnesses the power of neuroplasticity to heal chronic pain. But what does it really mean to reprocess pain? *Reprocessing* refers to the intentional reshaping of neural pathways associated with pain perception—in other words, changing the way your brain understands and relates to painful sensations. This may involve altering the interpretation of sensory signals, challenging automatic negative thoughts related to pain, and fostering new, healthier responses to pain sensations. Over time, using these tools to change the way the brain responds to painful sensations has the power to make those very sensations less painful and in many cases to eliminate the pain altogether.

As a typical example of the brain misinterpreting a sensation, imagine waking up in the morning with a dull pain in your head. You cannot help but dread the idea of having to get out of bed. Frustrated and in pain, you refuse to get up, fearing that starting your day will only make the pain worse. Without realizing it, you fall back asleep. Then alert! You flail out of bed forty-five minutes later realizing you overslept and will have to rush. Now you are not only in pain, frustrated, and anxious, but also late and not able to get your breakfast in. For the rest of the day, all your brain can do is focus on having started your day this way and the steadily increasing sensation of pain in your head. The headache gets worse as your day goes on, and your mood continues to dip. This cycle of pain, frustration, and worry is familiar to you—it feels like it's happening more and more often. It makes you worry. *Am I lacking certain vitamins? Do I have a food sensitivity I don't know about? Maybe my neck is out of whack and I need to get it adjusted? Or maybe it's something more serious, like a brain tumor?* Given your current view that pain is a signal of something wrong in the body, all of these are understandable associations to make.

However, you're missing one key component: the sensation of pain in your head as soon as you wake up. There is a core belief here that the painful sensation in your head is bad. Of course, there's a grain of truth in there: head pain sure does feel *unpleasant.* But the pain is not necessarily a signal of something wrong with your body, and there is more to the story than you think. Your brain is habitually interpreting the painful sensation in your head as dangerous, and not just a sign of physical danger but also a sign of other kinds of danger, like the threat that the headache poses to your ability to perform at work. The more you *reprocess pain*—the more you come to see it as a sensation rather than as a "problem" that must be fixed—the better chance you have of easing your way into the day in a way that might actually lead the pain to decrease or go away altogether.

In other words, if you can learn to view pain as simply a sensation—rather than a problem that needs to go away—you'll be operating from a place of safety, which, in turn, will make the pain and its consequences easier to deal with. Operating from a place of threat, on the other hand, can entrench the pain further and make it an even bigger problem to surmount than it would otherwise be. The goal here is to learn how to work with your nervous system, not against it. To begin exploring your relationship with perceptions of danger, take a moment to answer the following questions.

What is one non-pain thing your brain interprets as dangerous, and why? For some, it might be spiders. For others, flying in an airplane. For others still, emotional vulnerability. What is it for you?

Do you respond to this thing as though it were dangerous? Or are you able to acknowledge what your brain is telling you, and then move on, without necessarily acting on the danger your brain is flagging? If the latter, what would it be like to respond to your chronic pain and the things that trigger it in the same way?

_____

_____

_____

_____

_____

_____

How to Use This Workbook

So now that you've learned the basic concept of PRT, it's time to talk about how you actually can use this workbook. First, a bit about the people behind it. We are two mental health therapists who have our own personal histories with chronic pain. We initially came to PRT for our own healing. Then, after experiencing its transformative impact on our own symptoms, we began to practice PRT with clients. While this workbook is rooted in core PRT principles, it is very much an expression of how each of us practices PRT with clients, and it includes lessons we have learned along the paths of our own recoveries.

We emphasize the importance of embracing a multidisciplinary model. Before diving into this process, it's advisable to seek evaluation from a medical professional well-versed in mind–body approaches. This step is crucial to rule out potentially serious physical diagnoses. To connect with a physician specializing in this perspective, you can refer to the additional resources at the end of the book. If, after a medical professional has ruled out serious physical diagnoses, you still feel the need for additional reassurance, consider these steps:

1. Check in regularly with your medical provider to ensure you're receiving the care you need to support your engagement with a mind–body approach to pain treatment.

2. Acknowledge any skepticism or uncertainty you have about the mind–body connection in regard to your own pain.

3. Without reaching any hard-and-fast conclusions about your own potential for recovery, give yourself permission to explore techniques focused on harnessing the mind–body connection to foster a new relationship with pain.

Throughout this process, you have the autonomy to decide what's right for you. The guidance offered in this workbook is not a directive to abandon medical care, stop medications, or disregard your primary care provider's advice for ongoing wellness. Instead, it's an exploration into what might help alleviate your pain when conventional methods have fallen short.

This workbook contains many exercises. As you work your way through them, you'll notice that some have a ★ next to them. This symbol is our way of marking those exercises that we encourage you to return to again and again throughout your recovery.

Lastly, you'll find various worksheets and guided meditations available for download at the website for this book, http://www.newharbinger.com/53769. You can also visit this website by using the QR code displayed on this page. As you read, look for the ▓ icon next to the exercise. It will indicate that a worksheet or guided meditation is available online for the exercise in question.

We hope you enjoy the enhanced learning experience toward pain recovery.

Outcome Independence

One core PRT concept worthy of exploration from the outset is *outcome independence*, or the importance of practicing the tools used in reprocessing work, independent of the outcome (Gordon and Ziv 2021). The goal is not to make the pain go away and never come back but to change the way in which you respond to pain when it arises. The sneaky truth? Learning to respond to pain in an outcome independent manner is what ultimately causes the pain to go away. Maybe not this instant but over the long term, this new way of relating to unpleasant sensations is the secret to deactivating pain pathways.

On the other hand, if making pain go away is the outcome you're set on, paradoxically, it'll make it that much harder to actually achieve. Understandably, you want out of pain. That is why you are here, starting this workbook. But the tighter you hold onto that goal, the further away it will be. We will explain more about why this is true in the next chapter, when we explore the neuroscientific underpinnings of chronic pain. But for now, suffice it to say that learning to relax your grip on the outcome is one of the best things you can do for your own recovery. Easier said than done, we know.

To better understand what this may look like in real life, consider one of the author's experience. Vanessa faced many challenges as she grappled with trying to guide others in their recovery while also trying to figure out how to recover from her own pain. When Vanessa sought advice from a fellow therapist named Sherry at the Pain Psychology Center, Sherry responded by sharing some wisdom her dad had passed down to her: the process of moving through life is like carrying a scoop of rice in the palm of your hand. It's a given that, as you're walking on your journey, some rice will fall. But clenching your fist tightly around the scoop of rice to protect it will only lead rice to fall out from between your fingers when it wouldn't have otherwise.

This wisdom, passed from Sherry's father to Sherry and then on to Vanessa, serves as a steadfast guide in facing life's challenges. It encourages letting go, trusting the unfolding process, and adjusting our response to symptoms. Vanessa applied this wisdom, easing her grip, and embracing uncertainties. Recovery is not about tightly controlling your pain; instead, it's about learning more about your pain so you can, over time, loosen your grip. We encourage you to navigate through this work with kindness and patience, even during tough moments. For now, as you begin to explore this new way of relating to your symptoms, we ask you to release your hold on any specific outcome and simply focus on moving through the practical steps in this workbook, one by one. .

Let's take a moment to check in. Imagine visiting an aquarium. You've entered a cool, dark blue room. This room is quiet, peaceful, and comforting. There is a tall glass wall, from floor to ceiling, that is at least two-feet thick. The sun beams down onto the big body of water from above the tank. The light is trickling in through the water, glittering down onto you as you walk deeper into the room. You find a cement bench and sit down on the cool surface, dropping your shoulders as you sit back and giving a deep exhale. This is your time to just observe. Observe what thoughts you are having. Observe what sensations you are experiencing. Observe what you hear around you. Observe what you feel like watching tonight after you finish dinner. Take this time to create some space between you and the urgency to dive into this workbook and make progress. And when you are ready, place your bookmark on this page or fold the corner, and close the book shut. Be that observer in the aquarium, and take three gentle inhalations and three gentle exhalations. And when you are finished, come back to this page.

Now that you've returned, take a moment to jot down what you observed. There are no right or wrong answers, only observations.

_____

_____

_____

_____

_____

_____

You did it. This is your first foray into mindfulness: the process of sitting back and simply observing without judgment, even if it's uncomfortable. From that mindful place, you are going to set the intention for this work. Keeping in mind all that you have read and reflected on so far, what is your intention for this work? What is the attitude that you want to carry with you as you make your way through this workbook?

_____

_____

_____

Identifying Personal Goals

Now that you have set your intention, let's focus on how your personal goals in this process can set you up to have the best outcome. Dr. David Clarke, president of the Psychophysiologic Disorders Association (PPDA), emphasizes the importance of joy in your routine—a sense of lightness, ease, and playfulness that everyone deserves. What are the light, fun, playful things that you want to get back to? Or maybe, for the first time? Here, we're not talking about getting back to a rigorous daily routine. What we have in mind are things that bring you joy. Maybe that's going for a walk on the beach, sitting through a movie with your loved one, or learning to make pasta by hand.

Name three things that motivate you to do this work.

1. _____

2. _____

3. _____

Let these be a North Star to guide you if and when the going gets tough.

Changing habits is hard! It does not always feel peaceful and easeful. Actually, it often feels very uncomfortable. While we are moving in the direction of greater ease in our lives, the path there can be anything but easy. This work is not intended to be enjoyable, per se. But the ultimate goal is to find more joy. At the beginning of this chapter, you read Clara's personal account of her struggles with chronic pain. The good news is that she achieved significant relief by reprocessing her pain at the Pain Psychology Center. Through this work, Clara realized that her intense frustration with pain was a barrier to achieving a pain-free state. Her frustration had fueled her habitual problem solving, as well as a lack of playfulness and ease in her life. In therapy, Clara learned to track sensations while holding the process loosely, coming to know and trust that uncertainty would not harm her. These efforts to relate to her pain differently and untangle the complicated threads of thoughts, feelings, and behaviors that primed her nervous system for pain helped her achieve the life she enjoys today. Though Clara's experience is inspiring, it's essential to recognize that no two paths are the same. As you move ahead, whatever shape your journey takes, may patience, persistence, and compassion light your way.

CHAPTER 2

How Pain Works

The first major step in your recovery journey—the step that makes reprocessing pain possible—is to understand what pain is and how it works. The goal of this chapter is to help you do just that.

All pain comes from the brain. If you touch a hot stove, sensory input will travel from your hand to your brain (*Hot!*), where your brain will interpret that sensory input (*Danger!*), and send a pain signal in response (*Ouch!*). Pain is the brain's way of alerting you to danger—in other words, pain is a danger signal.

Whenever you feel pain in the body, it's because specific nerve fibers in your brain have been activated—when you burn your hand, it *feels* like the pain is coming from your hand, but the sensation is actually coming from the part of your brain that makes you feel pain in your hand. If a brain surgeon tickled that same part of your brain in just the right way, even in the absence of anything actually happening to your hand, you'd feel pain in your hand. Even if someone has lost their hand to amputation, stimulating that same part of the brain will cause them to feel the very same hand pain. This is what we mean when we say that *all pain comes from the brain*.

EXERCISE: Identifying Your Hot Spots

As shown in the diagram, different parts of your brain correspond to different parts of your body. When nerve fibers in the part of your brain corresponding to "tongue" are stimulated, you feel something in your tongue. When nerve fibers in the "thumb" part of your brain are stimulated, you feel something in your thumb. And so on.

Take a look at the diagram and circle the parts of your brain shown here that have been stimulated over the course of your own experience with chronic pain. Now take a colored pen and select your top three hot spots—that is, the three areas in your body where pain has been the most problematic—which in turn will reveal the three areas in the part of your brain shown here that have been the most stimulated.

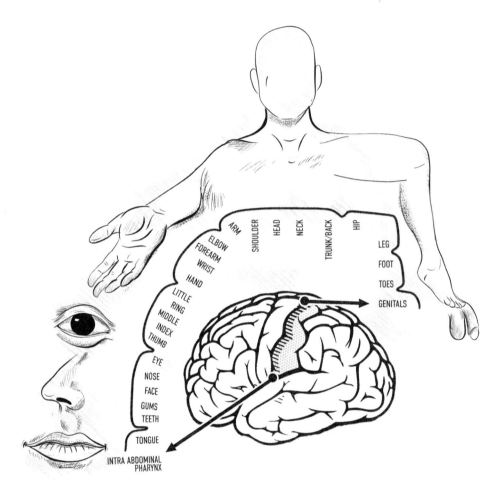

Figure 2.1 Somatosensory Cortex

The next time that you experience a chronic pain symptom—which could be right now as you read this very sentence—take a moment to think of this diagram and bring to mind the part of your brain that's being stimulated. Reflect on the fact that while you *feel* the pain in your body, the pain is actually coming from your brain. How does this reflection affect the way you think about your pain? Does this new understanding change your experience of the pain in any way? There are no right or wrong answers to these questions—your only task is to take some time to sit with them, and to be curious about what you find.

When the Brain Makes Mistakes

Ideally, the brain would only send a pain signal when there is actual danger, like when you burn your hand on the stove. But sometimes the brain makes mistakes. Although pain often represents genuine danger, sometimes the pain is real but the danger isn't. Your brain is more worried about keeping you safe than it is about getting it right.

Consider this case: A twenty-nine-year-old construction worker jumped onto a plank at a job site, causing a nail to pass all the way through his boot from one end to the other (Fisher, Hassan, and O'Connor 1995). In terrible pain, the construction worker was rushed to the hospital where he was sedated so the doctors could attend to his foot. When they were finally able to remove his boot, the doctors discovered that, in fact, the nail hadn't damaged his foot at all—it had passed right between his toes. And yet, in spite of there being no damage whatsoever, the man had experienced excruciating pain. Seeing the gruesome image of the nail passing through his boot caused his brain to send an alarm signal (*Ouch!*), even though there was no actual danger. In other words, the very real pain that the construction worker felt was a false alarm.

Now consider the scientific study in which a group of people were told that they would be hooked up to a machine that would deliver an electric current and cause a headache (Bayer, Baer, and Early 1991). Half of participants reported that they experienced pain in response to the electric current. The truth? There was no electric current. The expectation of pain was enough to cause their brains to sound the alarm, even though there was no actual danger.

In another study, research subjects experienced a simulated car crash. There was no actual impact, but through the magic of special effects, the subjects believed they had been rear-ended (Castro et al. 2001). Even though they only *believed* there had been impact, approximately 20 percent of the study's participants went on to develop *real* symptoms of whiplash. Their beliefs caused their brains to send a danger signal in the form of neck and back pain, even though nothing dangerous had actually occurred.

In all of these examples, there was some experience that primed the brain for pain. Even though there was no actual danger, the brain responded as if there were—the danger was false, but the pain was very real.

False Danger, True Pain

It may be tempting to chuckle at these stories, but the truth is it could happen to any of us. Our brains are great at lots of things, but telling the difference between true and false danger isn't necessarily one of them.

The brain often takes a better-safe-than-sorry attitude to danger, and as a result, it's quite possible that we'd experience the same excruciating pain as the construction worker if we saw a nail go through our boot or the same headache as the test subjects if we had electrodes hooked up to our scalps. In fact, if you're reading this book, it's likely that—just like the two of us—you've experienced your own version of false danger, true pain many times. And—just like us—understanding that true pain doesn't necessarily indicate real danger will open the door to your recovery.

The Brain on High Alert

It turns out that certain kinds of experiences can make the brain more likely to mistake a safe input for a dangerous one and send a false alarm in response. What these experiences have in common is they put the brain on high alert for signs of potential danger—they introduce an aspect of *fear*. The construction worker's horror upon seeing the nail go through his boot? A form of fear. The test subjects' trepidation about a forthcoming headache? Fear again. The participants' concern about the physical consequences of being rear-ended when they were in the whiplash simulator? You guessed it, fear.

Fear puts our brains on high alert—it puts us on guard. In psychology, the word for this high alert state is *hypervigilance*. Because the fearful brain is so preoccupied with protecting us from danger, it takes on even more of a better-safe-than-sorry attitude than it normally would—the fearful brain would always rather err on the side of caution. The problem is that when fear causes the brain to err on the side of caution, it makes it far more likely that neutral inputs will be mistaken for dangerous ones.

The Fearful Brain

Imagine that you're on a camping trip and you just learned that, not long ago, there was a bear attack nearby. You're walking alone through the forest near your campsite when you see a dark shadowy figure in the distance. Your brain shouts *Bear!*, your heart pounds, and your natural instinct is to run in the other direction.

If you believe the danger message that your brain is sending, you won't stick around long enough to see that the shadowy figure isn't a bear at all but is just a great big stump. When fear causes us to look at the world through a lens of danger, our perception becomes distorted. Furthermore, in the same way that fear can distort your visual perception, making your brain more likely to mistake safe stimuli (stumps) for dangerous ones (bears), fear can also distort your perception of physical sensations, making your brain more likely to mistake perfectly neutral sensations for dangerous ones. And, in the realm of physical sensation, what does the brain do when it perceives danger? That's right, it sends a pain signal to alert us! In this way, fear is the secret ingredient that causes us to feel very real pain even when there's no actual danger.

By causing the brain to err on the side of caution, fear makes the brain more likely to mistake safe sensations for dangerous ones, resulting in very real pain. Naturally, we begin to fear the pain itself, not only because of how much the pain hurts but also because of all the various ways that the pain impacts our lives. The more we fear the pain, the more sensitive the brain becomes to potential signs of danger, causing the brain to err even more on the side of caution than it did before, which ultimately causes us to feel even more pain. In this way, pain causes fear, which causes more pain, which causes more fear…and so on. In this phenomenon known as the *pain–fear cycle*, fear is the fuel that keeps pain burning (Gordon and Ziv 2021).

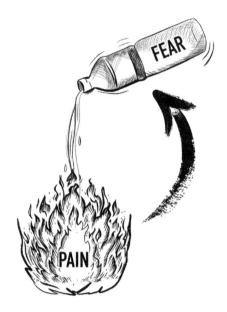

Figure 2.2 Pain–Fear Cycle

★ **EXERCISE:** Flavors of Fear

Fear is kind of like ice cream. It comes in many different flavors. Some ice cream flavors don't sound like ice cream at all (Rocky Road? Moose Tracks? Phish Food?), but upon closer inspection...yup, they're ice cream! Fear is the same way: it comes in many different forms, some of which might not seem like fear at first glance. But what all flavors of fear have in common is that they put the brain on high alert, causing the nervous systems to be extra sensitive to potential signs of danger.

The following chart shows different flavors of fear that people may experience surrounding their pain, as this fear manifests in their thoughts, feelings, and behaviors. Looking at the chart, place a check mark next to the thoughts, feelings, and behaviors that are familiar to you from your own experience. In the blank spaces, write down any other flavors of fear that you have experienced. In your daily life, continue to notice what flavors of fear emerge, and keep coming back to this page to update it as you move through the workbook.

Thoughts	Feelings	Behaviors
What if this pain means I have cancer or I'm seriously ill?	Tension	*Fixating* on the pain, that is, watching it like a hawk
Is the pain back? Is it getting worse? Is it getting better?	Anxiety	*Checking* to see if the pain is there...getting worse... getting better
I need another MRI, expert opinion, etc.	Uneasiness	*Preoccupation* with the pain and how it's affecting you
If the pain doesn't get better, I won't be able to...	Irritation	*Trying to control* the pain or make it go away (outcome dependence)
I hate my body!	Frustration	*Bracing* for the pain
I can't handle this.	Resistance	*Avoiding* activities that trigger pain
What am I going to do if the pain never ends?!	Anguish	*Complaining* about the pain and your inability to fix it
I'm never going to feel good again...	Despair	*Resigning* yourself to a life of suffering
I give up.	Dissociation	*Numbing out* with drugs, alcohol, food, TV, etc.

Working with Fear

For many, learning about the key role that fear plays in perpetuating pain can be overwhelming: *At first, I thought all I had to worry about was the pain, but now I have to worry about worry, too?* However, you've already done the hardest part: recognizing the ways that fear shows up in your own experience means that chronic pain's secret ingredient isn't so secret anymore. Once you begin to understand the relationship between fear and pain in your own life, you can also start to work with it, and that's where the magic happens. At this point, your job is to not allow the fear to slip back into secret ingredient territory. When fear emerges, shine a light on it and see it clearly for what it is.

In the days and weeks ahead, continue practicing being aware of how fear shows up in your own experience. Pay attention to fear that's specifically about the pain, but look out for other kinds of fear as well, because all fear puts the brain on high alert. Fear doesn't have to be *about* your pain to fuel it. Remember that your job is not to control fear or make it go away. Your only job is to notice it when it arises. Eventually, as you work through the chapters of this book, the fear will start to fade on its own—we promise. For now, when you notice that a flavor of fear has arisen in your body or mind, just notice it. You might even practice silently saying to it, *Hi fear, I seeeeee you!* as if the two of you were playing a lighthearted game of hide-and-seek. Remember, fear is not your enemy. In fact, it wants nothing more than to protect you—it just happens to be extremely confused about how to do that. Every time that you're able to see fear and respond to it in this lighthearted way, you take another step in the direction of breaking the pain–fear cycle once and for all.

So now you understand that pain is a danger signal sent by the brain to alert us to danger. And you also understand that sometimes the brain makes mistakes by interpreting safe inputs as dangerous and sending a very real pain signal even when there's no actual danger. When this kind of pain happens repeatedly, it's known as *neuroplastic pain* (Gordon and Ziv 2021).

Neuroplastic Pain and Other Symptoms

You can think of neuroplastic pain as the brain's version of a glitchy car alarm. If a car alarm is working properly, when does it go off? When someone is trying to break in, of course! But you've probably encountered a few car alarms in your life that weren't working quite right—you know, the kind that goes off whenever someone brushes up against the door or a truck drives by blasting loud music or a pigeon flies overhead. For those of us who experience neuroplastic pain, the brain habitually misinterprets neutral inputs as dangerous and sends a pain signal in response. Over and over and over again.

Some simple car alarms only have one sound that they repeat over and over to get your attention—honk, honk, honk. But fancy car alarms have a bunch of sounds they'll use to try and get your attention—honk honk, beep beep, weh weh, ding ding. The brain is like that fancy car alarm. It has a variety of alarms that it can use to signal danger, and pain is just one of them. Some of the brain's favorite danger signals include pain, anxiety, digestive issues, fatigue, dizziness, and itching. Although we mostly talk about pain in this book, you may be familiar with some of the brain's other danger signals. The good news? They all work pretty much the same way, and the information that we're giving you about pain also applies to these other symptoms.

Neural Pathways and Neuroplasticity

Why do we call this kind of pain "neuroplastic"? *Neuroplasticity* describes the changeability of the brain: "neuro" means relating to the nervous system, and "plastic" means easily shaped or molded. When we talk about neuroplasticity, what we're referring to is the way that the brain is changeable. Neuroplasticity isn't necessarily a good thing or a bad thing. It simply describes the way in which brains easily pick up new habits—habits that can be helpful or unhelpful. Neuroplastic pain just so happens to be one particularly unhelpful habit.

Imagine two forest trails: one is a big wide trail that is smooth and open from the many feet that have walked it before, and the other is a tiny trail that is so filled with roots, rocks, and undergrowth that it's hard to distinguish from the surrounding forest. If you were in the middle of a hike through the woods and had to choose between taking the big wide trail or the tiny overgrown one, you'd probably choose the big wide one. In fact, the big wide trail is not only easier to walk down but also so well-established that you might just walk down it without even realizing that the tiny overgrown trail is an option.

The brain's neural pathways are like this: the more a neural pathway is traveled, the smoother and wider it gets, and the easier and more automatic it becomes for us to travel down in the future. Conversely, the less we use a particular neural pathway, the more overgrown it will become, and the less automatically we'll end up using it in the future. In this way, the brain changes over time—the phenomenon called neuroplasticity.

Take a moment to think back on something you intentionally learned to do when you were younger—like tying your shoes, playing a song on the piano, executing a tricky dance move, or throwing a frisbee. Write down the name of the activity you recall:

_____

Remember how hard it was at the beginning? You likely stumbled for a while, awkwardly struggling your way through from one moment to the next. But at some point, you kind of started to get the hang of it. Then before you knew it, it was actually easy. And now? Maybe now you're able to do the thing perfectly without thinking about it at all. The more you practiced it, the more you traveled that trail through the forest in your brain, making it smoother and wider with each repetition. In other words, the more you practiced it, the more you *strengthened* that neural pathway, making the action easier and easier to do. This is an example of neuroplasticity.

And just as your brain can learn how to tie shoelaces or throw a frisbee, your brain can learn pain—and unlearn it.

How Pain Becomes Chronic

Unlike learning a new dance move, pain is not something that we learn on purpose. But whenever we respond to pain with fear, that's exactly what we're doing: practicing the pain–fear cycle and ensuring that the pain will persist. This is how the pain–fear cycle builds momentum in the brain and how pain becomes chronic.

At first, the pain might just be a tiny trail through the woods—a headache that you got one time during a particularly stressful period at work. But then you start to worry about getting another headache and how that would make it difficult to meet your upcoming deadline, and the prospect of missing a deadline really stresses you out…and then you get another headache. And now it's happened twice, and you feel like you really can't afford to get another one, because if you do, it will definitely start to affect your job performance… and then you get another headache. And so on, until before you know it, the pain–fear cycle is like a freeway running through the forest of your brain—the habit is so strong that it starts to happen automatically—and you've got chronic pain.

But what about chronic pain that begins with an injury? In that case, there is genuine physical danger at the outset, and that's what triggers the pain at first. And, as part of the nervous system's built-in protection mechanism, pain pathways can become hypersensitive in the wake of an injury to prevent you from injuring yourself further. But for many of us, this hypersensitivity persists long after it's served its purpose, causing us to continue experiencing pain even after the injury has healed. As the brain sends the pain signal repeatedly over time—accompanied by all the flavors of fear that would naturally accompany an injury—the pain-fear cycle becomes more deeply ingrained in the brain, causing the pain switch to become stuck in the on position. You end up with a pain-fear cycle highway, and the result is pain that persists long after the initial injury has healed and the genuine danger has passed.

A similar phenomenon occurs when there is an enduring structural issue in the body—for example, arthritis or a herniated disc—and the brain overreacts, treating it as extremely dangerous even though the actual danger level is mild or even nonexistent. As a result of this overreaction, you experience far more pain than necessary. Pain that could simply be a dull and barely noticeable ache is instead a volcanic eruption of physical suffering. Why? Because the pain-fear cycle has taken root. Once a flavor of fear enters the picture—even one as seemingly harmless as annoyance or irritation—the brain's hypersensitivity to potential signs of danger will increase, and we're off to the races. As this pattern is repeated over time, the pain-fear cycle becomes your brain's default state, and you've got chronic pain.

What all these varieties of persistent pain have in common is that most—if not all—of physical suffering is caused by the brain's hypersensitivity rather than a problem in the body. To return to the glitchy car alarm, the problem there isn't with the pedestrian brushing up against the car or the pigeon flying overhead—the problem is with the alarm, which is so sensitive to potential signs of danger that it can't tell the difference between a harmless passerby and a genuine threat. Similarly, the remedy to neuroplastic pain isn't found in surgery or medication that aims to fix a problem in the body—the remedy is found in rewiring the nervous system.

What's in a Name?

You might notice that there are a lot of different names out there for what is essentially the phenomenon that we refer to as "neuroplastic pain." As you explore this topic elsewhere—whether with your health care providers, in other books you read, or in online resources—you might come across other terms, such as nociplastic pain, central sensitization pain, mind–body syndrome, primary chronic pain, central pain syndrome, tension myositis syndrome (TMS), neural circuit disorder, and psychophysiologic disorder. While these terms may mean slightly different things on a technical level, for our purposes, they are interchangeable and you can think of all of them as different ways of saying "neuroplastic pain."

A Different Solution

Researchers at Northwestern University compared the brain activity of subjects who had experienced back pain for less than two months ("early back pain" group) to the brain activity of subjects who had lived with back pain for over ten years ("chronic back pain" group) (Hashmi et al. 2013). They found that the back pain–related brain activity in the early back pain group was limited to regions of the brain involved in acute pain, whereas back pain–related brain activity in the chronic back pain group was confined to a completely different part of the brain, which is associated with emotion-related circuitry.

The researchers followed the early back pain group for another year, comparing brain activity of those who recovered from their back pain to the brain activity of those who didn't. Among those who recovered, back pain–related brain activity diminished in time, whereas among those for whom the pain persisted, back pain–related brain activity decreased in the acute pain regions of the brain but increased in the regions associated with emotion-related circuitry.

The researchers observed that the brain activity of chronic pain sufferers was visibly different from the brain activity of those experiencing acute pain. What this tells us is that chronic pain happens via different neural pathways than acute pain, even though the two types of pain may *feel* the same. Chronic pain is not simply a version of acute pain that happens repeatedly over a long period of time—chronic pain is a completely distinct neural phenomenon.

So, given that chronic pain is different from acute pain, how can we treat it? We treat acute pain by working with the body—surgery, medication, and other physical interventions. But as you may know from your own experience, those physical interventions don't work so well when it comes to chronic pain. Why? Because it's a completely different problem, and a different problem that requires a different solution. The first step is getting curious about what's happening in your own nervous system.

Understanding vs. Believing

It's one thing to understand what neuroplastic pain is, and quite another to believe that some portion of your own pain is neuroplastic. The problem is that as long as you continue to believe that there is something seriously wrong with your body, that belief will continue to fuel the pain–fear cycle.

Luckily, you don't need to force yourself to believe that your own pain is neuroplastic—in fact, trying to force it can sometimes make the fear response more intense. Instead, your job is simply to be *open* to the information being offered and *curious* about the extent to which it resonates with your own experience. Keep this in mind as you engage with the following exercise.

EXERCISE: Self-Assessment

All pain is real and *feels* like it's coming from the body. For this reason, there's no way to tell whether pain is neuroplastic from the sensation alone. But, fortunately, as Alan Gordon lays out in his book *The Way Out*, there are certain signs you can look for that point to neuroplastic pain (Gordon and Ziv 2021). We've paraphrased his list here. As you review it, keep in mind that hardly anybody has *all* of these signs. If even a few of them resonate with you, then that's strong evidence that you experience neuroplastic pain.

As you review the list of signs, try to hold off on reaching any big conclusions one way or another about your own pain. Instead, remain as open as possible to the information you're reading and as curious as you can be about the ways that it might relate to your own experience.

_____ Your pain originated during a time of stress and/or worsens in the presence of stress.

_____ Your pain began with an injury but stayed much longer than it normally takes for that kind of injury to heal.

_____ Your pain began with an injury but then went away for a period only to reemerge sometime later.

_____ Your pain originated in the absence of any clear injury.

_____ Your symptoms are inconsistent—sometimes a particular trigger causes pain, and sometimes it doesn't. (For example, you always have pain when you do a particular activity, but sometimes it's mild and sometimes it's more severe. Or you have pain when you do one activity but significantly less pain when you do a very similar activity. Or you have pain only in certain contexts—at home but not on vacation, on weekdays but not on weekends.)

_____ You have a large number of symptoms. This can include pain in different parts of your body or a combination of pain and other symptoms such as anxiety, digestive issues, fatigue, dizziness, or itching. (While it is unlikely to have several unrelated physical conditions, a more likely explanation is that these conditions all share a common cause—an overprotective nervous system.)

_____ Your symptoms spread or move from one area or part of your body to another. (This is not how structurally caused pain typically behaves.)

_____ Your symptoms are triggered or worsened by stress. (The reverse can also be true— you may find that when you are engaged in a pleasurable activity and enjoying yourself, your pain decreases.)

_____ Your pain is triggered or worsened by things that have nothing to do with the structure of your body, including but not limited to the weather, sounds, smells, time of day, time of year.

_____ Your symptoms are symmetrical, so you have pain in the same part of your body but on opposite sides—both shoulders, both feet, both wrists. (Developing a physical problem on both sides of your body at the same time is very unlikely.)

_____ Your pain tends to come on *after* you complete an activity—walking, hiking, running, etc. (This delayed onset is not something that you see when pain is caused by structural issues in the body.)

_____ You have one or more of the following personality traits: perfectionism, conscientiousness, people pleasing, anxiousness.

_____ Your medical providers have not been able to agree on a clear structural explanation for your pain.

_____ You experienced adversity in childhood.

Once you've read through all the signs, go back and place a check mark next to those that resonate with your own experience.

All of the above can be signs of neuroplastic pain. Adversity in childhood is one that we will explore in more detail in the next chapter, so if you are curious whether this applies to you, stay tuned.

A Note About Medical Diagnoses

Although some people with neuroplastic pain have never been offered a clear medical explanation for their pain, many have. Indeed, if you have received a medical diagnosis, your pain can still be neuroplastic.

Certain medical diagnoses—like central sensitization syndrome, fibromyalgia, complex regional pain syndrome, interstitial cystitis, and chronic migraine—essentially mean "pain without a clear structural cause." In other words, they describe real pain that is unrelated to actual danger in the body. Increasingly, many medical providers think of these diagnoses simply as types of neuroplastic pain.

Some other diagnoses are intended to offer structural explanations for pain but don't do a very convincing job. Many people who experience chronic back pain have had an MRI or other scan done of their back, showing various "abnormalities" that doctors then point to as an explanation for the pain. But recent research has shown that these types of scans are not actually accurate indicators of pain. In one study, researchers evaluated MRIs from three thousand people with no symptoms of back pain (Brinjikji et al. 2015). Among twenty-year-olds without back pain, 37 percent had disc degeneration and 30 percent had disc bulges. Among eighty-year-olds without back pain, 96 percent had disc degeneration and 84 percent had disc bulges. What this research shows is that these so-called abnormalities are actually quite normal consequences of the aging process and are unreliable indicators of whether someone is going to be in pain or not. One study found that even among people with back pain, MRI abnormalities had absolutely no correlation with pain symptoms (Steffens et al. 2014). Although doctors mean well when they respond to a patient's complaints of back pain by pointing to abnormalities in the MRI, science tells us that this is unlikely to be the whole story.

Of course, some chronic pain is caused by structural issues in the body. Some examples include osteoarthritis, diabetic neuropathy, and certain autoimmune diseases like lupus. But even when there is a genuine structural issue at play, neuroplastic pain is often also along for the ride. Take osteoarthritis, for example. It's not uncommon for two people to experience similar degrees of joint degeneration but very different pain levels. One person is nearly incapacitated by the severity of their pain while the other barely notices any discomfort. Why? The first person's arthritis symptoms are amplified by neuroplastic pain: the overprotective nervous system is responding to a relatively minor issue as if it were a major threat. The second person's brain, on the other hand, is accurately assessing the situation and sending a pain signal that's proportional to the minimal degree of danger posed.

So, if you have received a medical diagnosis, don't throw away this book just yet. If other elements of the self-assessment resonated with you, there is a good chance that neuroplastic pain is playing a role in your symptoms and that the skills you will gain in this book are exactly what you need to find relief.

What was it like for you to complete the self-assessment? In our experience, some people who identify with multiple signs of neuroplastic pain are quick to believe that their own pain is neuroplastic, while others are slower to do so. While there are many reasons someone might be reluctant to accept the idea of their own pain being neuroplastic, one of the biggest obstacles to acceptance lies in the many myths that surround neuroplastic pain. Perhaps the most problematic of all is the myth that neuroplastic pain is "all in your head." So we want to say clearly, once and for all, that neuroplastic pain is *real* pain! Yes, neuroplastic pain—like all pain—comes from the brain. But that does not mean that it's fake or made up. While the danger may be false, the pain is as real as it gets.

EXERCISE: Confronting Common Myths

Let's take a moment to look at some of the myths chronic pain sufferers often hear about their symptoms. Read through the list, and then take a few moments to add any of your own that aren't already included.

"It's all in your head."

"Your pain isn't real."

"You're just too sensitive."

"You just have a low pain tolerance."

"You're weak."

"You just need to toughen up."

"Your pain is your own fault."

"You're broken."

"You're choosing to suffer."

"You're crazy."

"You're just looking for attention."

_____

_____

_____

Next, take a black pen or marker and go down the list, crossing each myth out one by one. You can do this however you like—one big line through it, zigzags, or writing the word "false" in big capital letters over the myth. Whatever method you choose, the point is to totally destroy it! Let all the anger and frustration you've felt over the years flow out of your pen, obliterating these myths on the page and in your own mind, once and for all.

Moving Forward

In this chapter, you've learned what pain is (one of the brain's favorite danger signals) and what it isn't (always a sign of real danger). You've come to understand the all-important role that fear plays in perpetuating neuroplastic pain. And, perhaps most importantly, you've become more aware of the role that flavors of fear play in your own experience of pain. This sets the stage for the work to come: changing your relationship with pain by untangling your relationship with the fear around the pain.

CHAPTER 3

The Overprotective Nervous System

In the last chapter, we uncovered the intricate dance between fear and pain. Now, we will unveil a side of your body's defense system that can be as frustrating as it is endearing. The overprotective nervous system is the body's equivalent of a helicopter parent. Exploring the life experiences that made your nervous system become overprotective will help you understand why an otherwise innocent stimulus can sometimes trigger a Code Red response from your nerves.

How the Nervous System Becomes Overprotective

Different life experiences—both big and small—can cause the nervous system to become overprotective. The result is a profound shift in how your nervous system perceives and responds to the world around you. It's as if the system had decided to upgrade to ultravigilant mode, ensuring your safety in the face of any potential danger, no matter how trivial it may seem. Your brain is like a not-so-careful librarian, shelving harmless events right alongside more serious ones in the "danger" section of your memory.

One type of experience that can kick your system up to ultravigilant mode is trauma. *Big T trauma* involves violence, abuse, severe neglect, the loss of a caregiver in childhood, or other serious threats to your physical safety. *Little t trauma* involves events that are not threats to your physical safety but still cause stress or endanger the mind. Little t trauma in childhood can be especially impactful. Maybe you grew up with an overly critical caregiver and felt you were never good enough, no matter how hard you tried. Or perhaps your caregiver struggled with mental health or substance use, and you felt like it was up to you to take care of them. Maybe your caregivers were so preoccupied with their own stress that you were left to attend to your own needs. Or maybe your home life was okay, but you were bullied at school or were involved in hypercompetitive academics or sports where you felt immense pressure to perform. In adulthood, little t trauma might take the shape of ongoing interpersonal conflicts, work stress, financial worries, legal trouble, or chronic health issues. Little t trauma can take countless forms, but what all these forms have in common is a tendency to make you perceive the world around you through a lens of danger.

Oftentimes, it's clear that experiences like ongoing violence or the death of a parent are a major trauma. And there are many resources, such as therapy, support groups, websites, and podcasts that focus on validating these incredibly painful experiences, which can provide healing and recovery. When it comes to little t trauma, however, we can often overlook it and forget that our nervous systems will be trained to respond to little t as if it were as significant as big T. Just like a not-so-careful librarian, your brain will shelve those little T events, often without you being aware of it, until they show up as a physical symptom of chronic pain.

Take your author Vanessa, for example. Vanessa endured many levels of trauma throughout her childhood, both big T and little t, growing up in a chaotic home and eventually being placed into foster care. Vanessa's brain normalized chaos as comfort in an effort to help her survive. Violence, abuse, feeling physically and emotionally unsafe at home and unable to tell anyone seemed to feel manageable as the great protector of her brain decided, "We cannot fight this, so in order to get through this, this has to feel normal to us." As a result, Vanessa became proficient in powering through, people pleasing, and smiling through the pain. However, later in life, she would begin experiencing symptoms of chronic pain. These symptoms would arise during high-pressure moments, such as navigating the hurdles of family relationships, making big life decisions, confronting career pressures, and even writing a workbook—all events that, while stressful, also seemed like part of regular life. Vanessa couldn't understand how seemingly small events would cause such physical distress, including chronic pelvic floor pain, migraines, hives, neck pain, chronic fatigue, and irritable bowel syndrome. Even with a 4.0 GPA, promotions, a loving relationship, and everyone cheering her on, it didn't feel like enough. It felt like in a split second, all of this could go away if she wasn't doing everything "right." It didn't make sense, logically, with Vanessa's big T childhood experiences in the background, that the path to a happier, safer life would feel so bad. What Vanessa didn't realize was that the stress from the things she was taking on—though leading to something great—was creating little t events for her nervous system, one after the next. Eventually, Vanessa began to understand what her overprotective nervous system was doing: it was telling her that it wasn't sure it felt safe, even when things seemed to be so.

We all have moments when our system interprets a breeze as a tornado, reacting with an intensity that seems disproportionate. This heightened vigilance is often born from an earnest intention: to shield you from perceived threats. It's a reflection of your system's commitment to safeguarding your well-being. We want to encourage you to delve into the underlying reasons why this happens to you—from minor incidents that echo through your neural pathways (like the anxiety that forces you awake throughout the night when you have a busy day ahead) to experiences of significant trauma and adversity. With empathy and insight, the following exercise invites you to shed light on how life's complexities have shaped your own responses.

EXERCISE: Understanding the Overprotective Nervous System

Take this moment to think about your own nervous system's response to experiences large and small, and ask yourself, *How is it understandable?* Use this question to compassionately, patiently ask how it makes sense that your nervous system would be stuck on the helicopter-parent setting. Whether it is a big T or little t, fill in the following bubbles, identifying experiences, situations, and memories that could explain why your nervous system is in a persistent state of Code Red. Be aware that if people who played a role in these experiences are still in your life, it may further intensify your nervous system's alarm signals.

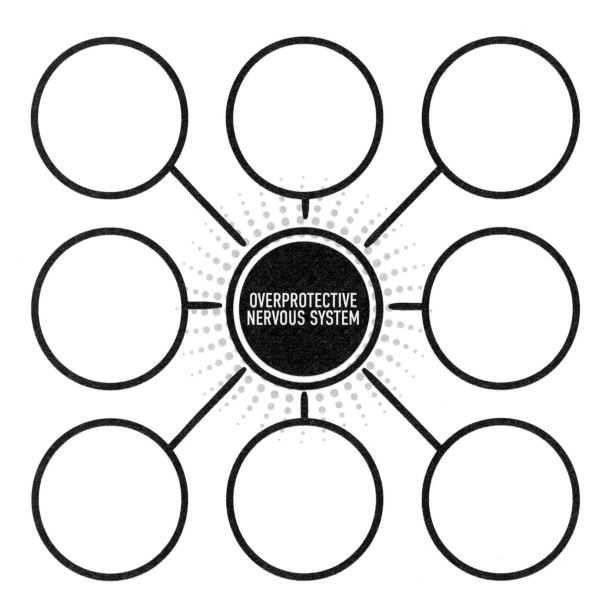

Figure 3.1 Overprotective Nervous System

Before continuing on to the next section, if you're feeling the need to take care of yourself after the work you put into the previous exercise, we encourage you to take some space. If you need to take a break, place a bookmark on this page and return when you're ready. You can get some fresh air, grab a glass of water, or listen to a song that promotes a mood that you would like to be in. This workbook is not a race. Remember to take care of yourself along the way.

If you find that revisiting these memories triggers flashbacks, panic attacks, dissociation, or other symptoms of extreme distress, we encourage you to consider seeking out a trained trauma therapist to support you with this component of the work. Please see the additional resources at the end of this workbook for information on how to get connected with a mental health professional.

Bringing Protective Traits into Balance

We develop protective traits as a natural response to the kinds of experiences you explored in the previous exercise. These are thought, feeling, and behavior patterns that emerge to keep us safe in the midst of both big T and little t traumas. Over time, protective traits can take on a momentum of their own, becoming our default modes for relating to the world, continuing to do their protective thing long after the original threat has passed. Although they originally emerged to protect us, in the long term, these traits can inadvertently cause us to suffer by fueling the pain–fear cycle, which is why we need to bring them into balance.

Read through the common protective traits below, placing a check mark next to those that feel familiar to you. If you have protective traits that aren't listed here, add them in the space provided.

Trait	Description
Urgency	Uncertainty can be uncomfortable for everyone, and it can be especially difficult with chronic pain: not knowing what's causing your pain, how to make it better, or if you'll ever recover. You understandably feel the need to find all the answers *now*, before anything worse happens. Unfortunately, this urgent pursuit of resolution validates the brain's belief that danger abounds, fueling even more pain.

Trait	Description
Bracing for impact	Bracing is a natural reflex that can keep you safe when a baseball flies at your face or a car is about to collide with yours. It makes sense that this same protective instinct leads you to brace against the impact of chronic pain itself and the many ways it affects your life. But tensing against the unknown reinforces the brain's belief that there is something dangerous to brace against, which intensifies your pain.
Powering through	Powering through stems from an understandable desire to keep going, no matter the obstacles. In practice, you might force yourself to stay late to get that last bit of work done, even though you're famished; to wait ten more minutes, even though you have to go to the bathroom; or just to keep walking through the pain. Unfortunately, the message this sends to your brain is that it needs to send louder signals to get your attention.
Problem solving	Solving problems can be both satisfying and empowering. But you can get stuck in fix-it mode, obsessively puzzling through problems and searching for solutions, which only serves to reinforce the idea that there is a problem to solve.
Intensity	Giving it your all. Going hard. Putting in 110 percent. Intensity can be an incredible source of strength and effectiveness. But when it becomes habitual, intensity signals to your nervous system that the obstacles you face are so massive that they require a turbocharged response—in other words, it reinforces the lens of danger.
Perfectionism	Perfectionism usually has a good reason to develop in the first place, such as to protect you from overly critical caregivers or to open academic or professional doors that would otherwise be closed. But when it becomes your default setting, perfectionism is like walking a tightrope without ever looking down: it feels like your life depends on it, even if you're actually only one foot off the ground.

Trait	Description
People pleasing	As social beings, we naturally want to please others. But this instinct can kick into overdrive, making you feel as though disappointing others would be a threat to your well-being. When that sense of threat is present, the brain is more likely to mistake neutral sensations for dangerous ones.
Conscientiousness	You may feel that it's up to you—and you alone—to make sure that things don't go awry. This trait often originates as a survival response to childhood stressors, such as unreliable caregivers or parentification. If you feel like everything rests on your shoulders, and carry the fear that slipping up or letting something fall through the cracks will lead to terrible consequences, this persistent sense of threat can put your nervous system on high alert.
Avoidance	We are hardwired to avoid that which causes pain. But when you habitually work to avoid discomfort, you inadvertently reinforce the brain's notion that discomfort itself is a threat to your safety, prompting your brain to become even more sensitive to potential signs of danger.
Rumination	Really thinking something through can be a powerful tool. But when the same thoughts play on a loop in your mind, they're no longer an avenue to insight. These can be thoughts that you wouldn't have this pain if only that one thing had happened differently, thoughts that you'll never get better, thoughts that you'll never be happy again. This kind of thinking turns up the fear dial, exacerbating pain symptoms.
Self-judgment	Self-judgment grows out of the natural inclination to do the best you can. But in the realm of chronic pain, trying to keep yourself on track by holding yourself to high standards, or speaking to yourself using harsh or punishing language, actually has the opposite effect.

Trait	Description
Control	In the midst of chaos, control can be a lifeline. But in the realm of chronic pain—which so often feels profoundly out of control—gripping tightly only serves to reinforce the brain's belief in a threat that needs containing.
Fragility	Chronic pain can make you feel fragile. Maybe a health care provider told you to be careful about how much you lift, to abide by a strict anti-inflammatory diet, or to be careful to "manage your stress." But by buying into the message that you're uniquely vulnerable, you validate your brain's view that you need to handle yourself with kid gloves *or else*.
Numbing	Pain and distress are unpleasant, so it makes sense that you would take steps to distance yourself from those experiences by turning to drugs, alcohol, food, binge-watching TV, and so on. But when you escape in this way, you reinforce the brain's belief that there's something inherently dangerous about discomfort.

A key to healing is learning to understand and relate to these protective traits differently. The goal is to enable these traits to come back into balance, and a therapeutic approach that we find particularly helpful is parts work. Parts work invites us to look at our inner world—all of the traits, patterns, and habits we see within us—as different parts of ourselves, each with different roles to play. Those of us with overprotective nervous systems tend to have multiple protective parts that are out of balance, working so hard to protect us that they can inadvertently cause other problems, like neuroplastic pain. You might have a part that braces for impact, another part hyperfocused on problem solving, and yet another part that does its very best to power through whatever challenge may arise. Or you might have a perfectionist part, a ruminating part, a people-pleasing part, or a controlling part. You might have a part that avoids anything anxiety-provoking, a part that criticizes you in its effort to keep you on the right track, or a part that numbs you out to give you some relief from life's challenges. Or you might have some combination of all of these—and maybe others that aren't listed here.

Your job is to get to know your protective parts so you can start working with them rather than against them. The following exercise—adapted from internal family systems (IFS), one parts work model that has informed our approach—will help you do just that. IFS, developed by Dr. Richard Schwartz, has been used to help chronic pain sufferers connect with and heal parts of themselves that were inadvertently driving their pain symptoms (Schubiner, Schwartz, and Siegel 2021). One IFS technique that we find particularly helpful involves communicating directly with protective parts, asking them questions to understand where they're coming from and what they're trying to do (Schwartz 2021; 2023). In this exercise, you'll have the opportunity to connect with your own protective parts.

★ EXERCISE: Getting to Know Your Inner Protectors

Choose one of your parts that works hard to keep you safe. If you're aware of a protective part that's already active at this moment, go with that; if not, choose one that feels particularly accessible to you. It can be any of the parts listed above or another protective part that we haven't named. Once you've identified the part you want to connect with, take some time to sit quietly and explore the questions below.

Can you feel this part in your body? If so, where do you feel it? Go ahead and bring your awareness there. Use a few words to describe how it feels.

_____

_____

Does this part have a name? For example, "the push-through part" or "the perfectionist part."
If a name doesn't come naturally, there's no need to force it. Feel free to move on, and if one
arises later, come back to fill this in.

_____

_____

When did this part first come into your life? How did it get its job?

_____

_____

_____

_____

What are some examples of times when this part successfully helped to protect you?

_____

_____

_____

_____

What does this part desire most deeply?

_____

_____

_____

_____

_____

What does this part fear would happen if it stopped doing its job?

_____

_____

_____

_____

Is there anything else this part wants you to know?

_____

_____

_____

Take a moment to reconnect with this part again by bringing your awareness to the place in your body where you feel it. Stay with it for a few moments and thank it for all that it's shared with you today. If it feels authentic to you, go ahead and thank it for all the ways that it has worked so hard to protect you. Let it know that although this may be the first time you're connecting with it, it won't be the last. There will be more opportunities to connect directly with your protective parts throughout this workbook and beyond.

Because most of us have more than one protective part that needs our attention, we encourage you to return to the exercise you just did again and again as needed, writing your answers on a separate piece of paper or in your journal. When you notice that a protective part is particularly activated, whether in relation to pain (worrying about what's causing the pain, tensing with frustration when pain arises, or working hard to avoid pain triggers) or otherwise (with perfectionism, people pleasing, conscientiousness), it's a valuable opportunity to get to know that part better. When this happens, take a few moments to sit quietly, return to this exercise, and connect.

Working with Your Protective Parts

Now that you've begun getting to know your protective parts, how do you begin to work with them rather than against them? When our protective parts are out of balance, it can feel like a crowded school bus without a driver—each part urgently struggling to grab the wheel in a frantic effort to keep the bus on course. But once you begin to relate to your parts in a curious, attentive way, suddenly the bus has a driver: you. As you get to know your parts, directly connecting with each, one by one, they will gradually relax enough to step into the passenger seats, allowing you to take the wheel.

Once you're in the driver's seat, you can intentionally call on other internal qualities to help bring your system into balance. So, if you notice that your problem-solving part is in hyper fix-it mode, you can connect with it directly by asking it questions, as you did in the last exercise. Once it feels seen and understood enough to relax its grip, you can explore inviting in other qualities that will help to harmonize your approach to the problem before you, such as patience, acceptance, and a willingness to explore new avenues. The art of balance involves honoring both your resilience and the wisdom of knowing when to pause.

As you navigate the landscape of chronic pain, think of your protective parts—and the traits they carry—as colors in your personal palette of resilience. They have helped keep you safe for so long, and by learning to turn toward them rather than struggling against them, you are inviting them back into balance.

Confusing Unpleasant with Bad

Another way the brain can be overprotective is a natural tendency to confuse pleasant and unpleasant with good and bad. Leaving this natural tendency unchecked can lead to some big mistakes. It's like eating loads of french fries—super pleasant but not so good from a nutrition standpoint. And while working out can feel pretty unpleasant sometimes, it's one of the best things you can do for your mental and physical health. Similarly, when the brain unquestioningly interprets an unpleasant sensation as *bad*—a sign of something wrong, dangerous, or otherwise threatening—we can run into some pretty big problems.

Picture this: your nerves with their tiny binoculars are scanning for danger as soon as you open your eyes in the morning. They land on something unpleasant: a twinge of head pain, that familiar ache in your back, or a feeling of heaviness in your limbs. And there it is, evidence of the danger your brain was looking for. But what if the unpleasant sensations your brain discovers are nothing more than that? Unpleasant doesn't necessarily mean *bad*—it might just mean unpleasant.

Referring back to Vanessa's story, we know that her childhood was less than ideal, but her future was looking bright. However, her brain habitually interpreted unpleasant as bad, associating the unpleasant—albeit comparatively mundane—career or relationship stress she faced later in life with the stress involved in being in a big T environment that was actually dangerous. If she woke up with unpleasant sensations of pain or fatigue, her brain would panic and dread the day as if there were something truly threatening looming ahead. In response, Vanessa's protective parts would kick into gear—she would lean into powering through, which would in turn lead to increased levels of people pleasing and perfectionism. And doing that eventually caused her nervous system to feel so overwhelmed that it created even more chronic pain symptoms as a way to call her to rest.

All brains have the natural tendency to interpret an unpleasant feeling as something bad. Overprotective nervous systems are even more likely to err on the side of caution than the average brain, and in this way, they're even more primed to misinterpret neutral signals as dangerous ones and to respond with pain or other alarm signals. So, the next time you experience an unpleasant sensation, consider the power of interpretation. Whether it's the burn of a physical workout or the sharp sensation when you stand up, your brain's filter determines the narrative. By distinguishing between pleasant and good as well as unpleasant and bad, you guide your brain to understand that not all that feels nice is beneficial, and not all that feels uncomfortable is detrimental. By nurturing this awareness, you're empowering yourself to make choices that align with your long-term well-being.

Pain and Conditioning

The concept of *conditioning* offers significant insight into how our brains respond to pain. The Russian psychologist Ivan Pavlov first discovered this aspect of how the brain works in his classic experiment with dogs. Here is how it went: A dog hears a bell ring just before being presented with food. Over time, the dog begins to associate the bell with the impending meal. As a result, even when food isn't immediately present, the dog salivates at the sound of the bell.

Now, let's apply this idea to pain responses. Our brains can associate certain cues or contexts with pain. If you've ever winced at the thought of a needle, it's likely because your brain has linked needles with pain from past experiences. Understanding conditioning helps us realize that our pain responses can be shaped by various factors—not just the raw physical inputs. Imagine someone who experienced pain during a specific activity, like bending over to tie their shoes. Over time, their brain might associate the bending motion with pain, even if the initial injury has healed.

The good news is that just as conditioning can create pain associations, it can also be used to reshape these connections. This is where strategies for reprocessing your pain come into play. By consciously altering your responses to pain-associated cues, you can recalibrate your brain's conditioned reactions.

The idea here is that your responses are not just about physical inputs but also about the associations the brain makes, which can be distorted. In this way, the pain you experience may result more from the association your brain has made among a variety of other factors, including thoughts, emotions, behaviors, and environmental cues, than anything structural in your body. By recognizing this process, you gain the tools to reshape your responses and establish a more empowered relationship with pain. As you navigate this terrain, envision yourself as the conductor of your mental responses, using the principle of conditioning to fine-tune and adjust your reactions to more skillfully support your own well-being.

Take an example from your author Olivia's life. Before learning about neuroplastic pain, Olivia had a long history of exertion headaches: more often than not, when she physically exerted herself in a way that caused her heart rate to increase for a sustained period, she would end up with a splitting headache that lasted for many hours. In light of this, she understandably believed that exercise gave her headaches and that the only way to prevent headaches was to avoid exercise. As a result, she largely avoided strenuous aerobic activity.

Even though she loved exercise, she didn't want to pay the price of the headache that would so often come with it.

Luckily, Olivia eventually learned about neuroplastic pain. Once she understood the relationship between fear and pain, she came to recognize the hidden role that fear was playing in perpetuating her headaches. She noted that if she even thought about going for a run, she'd often start to worry about the headache that might follow. And if she actually did go running, the flavors of fear would start popping up like fresh popcorn at a busy cinema! She'd worry about when a headache might start, how bad it could get, and how it might interfere with the rest of her day. She'd start to feel anxious and vulnerable. And as she noticed her heart rate picking up, she would obsessively check the sensations in her head to see if the pain had begun, and if so, how bad it was.

For Olivia, aerobic exercise was a trigger launching her overprotective nervous system into high gear. Once she was armed with an understanding of the pain–fear cycle, however, Olivia came to see that aerobic exercise wasn't actually causing her headaches. Rather, it was her brain's fearful response to exercise that was truly causing her pain. For Olivia, getting to know her own overprotective nervous system in this way held the key to her recovery.

Before you learned about neuroplastic pain, you believed that your triggers caused your pain, but now you understand that it's not quite that simple. Fear is the secret ingredient that transforms something from an otherwise harmless experience into a trigger. In this next exercise, you'll have the opportunity to map the route that your brain takes on its journey from trigger to pain.

EXERCISE: Pain Maps

In the first column, identify a trigger that you've always believed caused you pain. This might be a behavior, like sitting, walking, or moving your body in a particular way. Or it might be an environmental factor, like a certain weather condition or a specific smell. It might be a kind of food or a category of foods. Or it might be something else altogether.

Next, in the third column, identify the symptom of pain that you associate with this trigger. Fill out the left and right columns for each trigger-symptom pair you can identify from your own life. Note: If you experience other physical symptoms, like itchiness, fatigue, nausea, or something else, this exercise is an opportunity to identify these symptoms and their corresponding triggers too.

Finally, in the center column, identify the flavors of fear that arise between triggers and symptoms. While you might be able to fill out this column from memory, we recommend that you take your time. Perhaps take a few days to pay attention to the precise thoughts, feelings, and behaviors that arise when you encounter one of these triggers in your daily life.

For guidance, Olivia's example of running appears first. For additional support filling out this section, turn back to the "Flavors of Fear" exercise in chapter 2.

Trigger	→	Flavors of Fear	→	Symptom
Olivia's example: *Running*	→	Thoughts: *Uh oh, I really don't want to get a headache.* Feelings: *Anxious, vulnerable* Behaviors: *Repeatedly checking sensations in head to see if pain has started*	→	*Headache*
	→	Thoughts: Feelings: Behaviors:	→	

Trigger	→	Flavors of Fear	→	Symptom
	→	Thoughts: Feelings: Behaviors:	→	
	→	Thoughts: Feelings: Behaviors:	→	
	→	Thoughts: Feelings: Behaviors:	→	

Trigger	→	Flavors of Fear	→	Symptom
	→	Thoughts: Feelings: Behaviors:	→	

Cultivating Self-Compassion

In your journey of self-discovery and healing, it's crucial to approach your overprotective nervous system with the gentleness and understanding you would extend to a dear friend. Your nervous system is that dedicated companion who means well but occasionally gets a tad bewildered about how to best support you. Think of it as a helper navigating a complex map with some missing pieces, and doing its utmost to guide you but sometimes taking detours and unexpected turns. This confusion arises not from an intention to cause distress but from an innate desire to ensure you're out of harm's way.

Now that you've come to understand your overprotective nervous system more deeply—why and how your protective parts do what they do—you can begin the process of integrating awareness of and compassion for your nervous system into your everyday life. Let's begin with a formal practice.

EXERCISE: Treating Your Nervous System with Kindness

In this practice, you will offer kindness toward your overprotective nervous system as if you were offering understanding to a friend going through a tough time. It's about acknowledging your system's efforts while gently guiding it toward a more balanced approach.

Step 1: Observation

Start by observing your body's reactions and responses in those moments when a protective part takes the driver's seat. Notice any shifts in your body, thoughts, or emotions. Is there a slight tightening, an anxious thought, or a surge of adrenaline? By becoming attuned to these signals, you're opening the door to understanding your protective part's presence.

Step 2: Validation

Remind yourself that your nervous system is acting from a place of concern. Validating its intention can help you cultivate patience and empathy toward its responses. You might say, *Hello, protector. I see you're here, watching out for me.* This simple acknowledgment creates a bridge of recognition, inviting a more conscious interaction with this aspect of yourself.

Step 3: Gentle Redirecting

Just as you might guide a concerned friend toward a more relaxed perspective, gently redirect your nervous system's focus. Rest your eyebrows, part your teeth, and reflect with a few natural breaths.

Step 4: Gratitude

Express gratitude for your nervous system's protective nature. Recognize that its vigilance has kept you out of harm's way on numerous occasions. Picture yourself extending a gentle hand and saying, "I understand you're trying to keep me safe, even if it feels overwhelming at times." This practice fosters a space of acceptance and validation, rather than unconsciousness or resistance, where growth can flourish. By noticing, greeting, and showing kindness to your protective part, you're forging a connection that nurtures understanding and healing, and fostering a loving dialogue within yourself.

Step 5: Self-Compassion

Treat yourself with the same kindness you're extending toward your nervous system. Understand that your responses are natural and that you're in the process of growth and learning.

After you complete this practice, you may want to write your reflections in your journal.

When you notice your nervous system going into high alert, pause for a moment. Instead of becoming frustrated, view it as an opportunity to understand its cues, and use the above practice to show compassion toward your overprotective nervous system.

When your overprotective nervous system is activated, you can also try following the four-step process we call NABS: notice, acknowledge, befriend, and shift.

1. *Notice* when your protective parts are at the wheel. Observe the shifts in your body, thoughts, or emotions that most typically mark your stress—say, a slight tightening, an anxious thought, a surge of adrenaline, or a bracing for pain.

2. *Acknowledge* that your protective part has kicked into gear. If, for example, your perfectionist part has shifted into gear, say to yourself: *Oh wow, there's perfectionism, working hard to make sure that I do this just right.*

3. *Befriend* your protective part by greeting it with curiosity and warmth. Take a moment to connect with its intention to protect you, and thank it for everything it has done and continues to do to try and keep you safe. Crucially, this doesn't mean you immediately do what your inner protector tells you to do. Rather, you're simply acknowledging that from the part's perspective, its protective response makes perfect sense.

4. *Shift* into a new gear. There's no need to get into a wrestling match with your protective part. Instead, practice kindness toward it, seeing if it would be willing to give you some space. If it accepts your invitation, then you can decide what you'll do next from a place of full awareness rather than fear, contraction, instinct, or reflex.

Take a picture of these steps or write them on a sticky note as a reminder when your protective parts try to take the wheel. And, if a part is unwilling to step back, respect that.

Take this as an opportunity to strengthen your relationship with that part, and get to know it better. Try returning to the "Getting to Know Your Inner Protectors" exercise, or you can simply bring your awareness to the place in your body where you feel that protective part and patiently stay present with it for some time, accepting it as it is without asking it to change or go away.

Learning to attend to your protective parts in this kind and gentle way is a crucial part of the rewiring process and, in the long run, will help your nervous system more accurately distinguish real threats from false alarms.

Moving Forward

With time and practice, you can develop a therapeutic partnership with your nervous system. As you navigate life's twists and turns, approach each interaction with the intention of understanding, patience, and kindness. Ask yourself, as you contemplate your inner protector's response to pain symptoms or stressful situations, *How is this understandable?* Then, speak to your nervous system as you would to that cherished friend, gently guiding it through moments of confusion and helping it recalibrate its responses.

This process will take work, and it won't always be easy or straightforward. But it will happen if you persist. Remember, too, that healing is not about silencing or suppressing parts of ourselves but is about fostering acceptance and nurturing growth. You're on a transformative journey, one that embraces your innate wisdom and invites healing from within. And you're fostering a harmonious partnership between your mind and body, which can lead to a more empowered approach to managing your experiences.

CHAPTER 4

Building a Foundation of Safety

In the last chapter, you began developing a new relationship with your overprotective nervous system, which will help you approach it with understanding and compassion. In this chapter, you will take this relationship a step further, building the foundation of safety that will make it possible to reprocess pain in the chapters to come.

If a pervasive sense of danger lies at the root of neuroplastic pain, what is the corresponding remedy? Perhaps not surprisingly, the remedy lies in safety, or the opposite of danger. The more familiar the nervous system becomes with safety, the less it will err on the side of caution, and as it begins to relax its better-safe-than-sorry approach, the less prone it will be to mistaking safe sensations for dangerous ones. Ultimately, our goal is to help the brain view sensations through a lens of safety rather than a lens of danger. Returning to an example from chapter 2, we want to help the brain recognize the stump for what it is—a stump—where it once saw a bear. If fear is the fuel that keeps pain burning, a sense of safety is the fire extinguisher that puts out the flames.

First, you will learn more about the foundation of safety you already have. Then you will learn new tools aimed at helping you think, feel, and behave in ways that will strengthen that foundation.

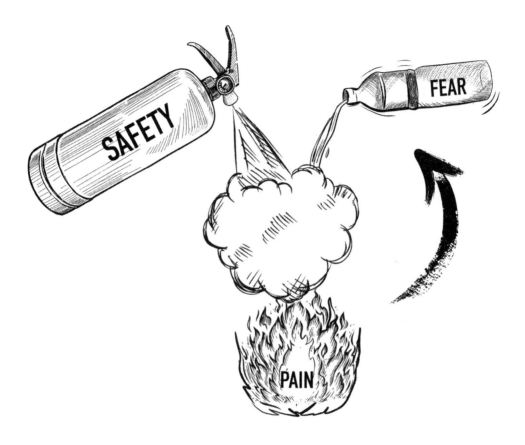

Figure 4.1 Interrupting the Pain–Fear Cycle

Getting to Know Your Safety Network

We've asked you to imagine that the brain is like a forest with each neural pathway like a trail in that forest. Now we want to add another concept. When different forest trails connect to each other to make a web of crisscrossing trails, they form a trail network. Similarly, for our purposes, when different neural pathways connect to each other, we can think of them as a *neural network*.

Although every human brain contains countless neural networks, what those neural networks look like from one brain to the next varies enormously depending in part on the kinds of experiences that the brain has had. To understand this better, let's imagine two different brains. The first brain belongs to a young man who was born and raised in Siberia. His neural network for *pineapple* is rather small: he's seen a few photos of pineapples, so he knows what they're called and he knows what they look like, but he's never actually touched, smelled, or tasted one in real life. Now, imagine a second brain that belongs to a young man who was born and raised in Hawaii. His neural network for *pineapple* is massive: it includes not only what pineapples are called and what they look like but also what they smell like, taste like, feel like, and how to tell when a pineapple is perfectly ripe, along with hundreds of memories involving pineapples, feelings associated with picking them fresh from his grandmother's garden, the complicated colonial history of pineapple farming, a long list of favorite pineapple recipes, the way his mouth feels when he's eaten one too many pieces of pineapple, images of elaborate sculptures carved to look like pineapples, and so on.

Similarly, each of us has a unique neural network for *safety*. How robust your own network is will depend on the kind of experiences you've had in your life so far. People who are very familiar with feeling safe are likely to have very robust neural networks, filled with memories, emotions, and other associations with safety: people around whom they feel or have felt safe, times they felt seen and cared for, places that help them feel grounded and stable. People who are very unfamiliar with feeling safe, including those who experienced persistent trauma in childhood, are more likely to have a relatively slim *safety* network, one that contains the concept of safety but lacks experiences, memories, and feelings associated with the concept.

In the spaces provided, take some time to map out what your own neural network for safety might look like. You may have a lot to write down or not much at all. Wherever you find yourself on this spectrum is okay. If you find it challenging to think of something to put in a particular box, feel free to leave it blank. There is no need to force anything. Think of this exercise as an opportunity to reflect on your real lived experience as it is.

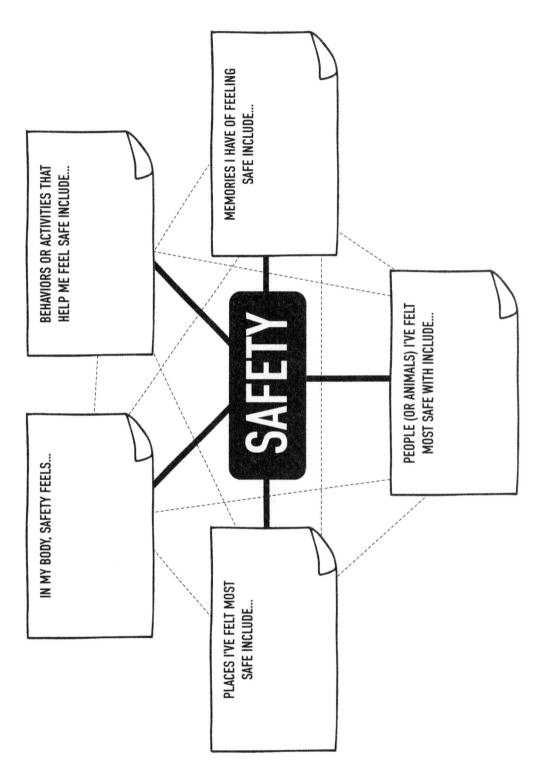

Figure 4.2 Mapping Your Safety Network

Many people reflecting on these questions will realize, perhaps for the first time, just how unfamiliar they are with feeling safe. If this is true for you, you may find that acknowledging this can be emotional. Whether you feel sadness, anger, grief, or something else altogether, your feelings are natural and understandable. Please take a moment to make space for whatever comes up. If you want to take a break to journal, go for a walk, snuggle your pet, or talk with a friend, we encourage you to do so. As we will discuss more in chapter 6, learning to acknowledge difficult feelings and make space for them is an important part of the healing process. When you are prepared to continue reading, come back to this point.

By practicing different thoughts, feelings, and behaviors, you can harness the power of neuroplasticity to strengthen your safety network. As your nervous system becomes more familiar with a sense of safety, it will gradually become less overprotective. There is no need to force this change to happen. Rather, it's a natural process that will unfold at its own pace. Your only job is to put one foot in front of the other and keep walking.

If you're already quite familiar with feeling safe, then the practices in this chapter will help you further develop your foundation of safety in preparation for the work ahead. If, on the other hand, you have not had much personal experience with feeling safe, then you may want to spend some additional time with these practices before moving on to the next chapter. You're also welcome to return to these practices whenever it feels helpful. The exercises offered here are lifelong tools for you to return to again and again whenever your nervous system needs soothing.

Strengthening Your Safety Network

Let's start by looking at three broad categories of human experience: thoughts, feelings, and behaviors. They are interconnected and are constantly influencing one another, as illustrated below.

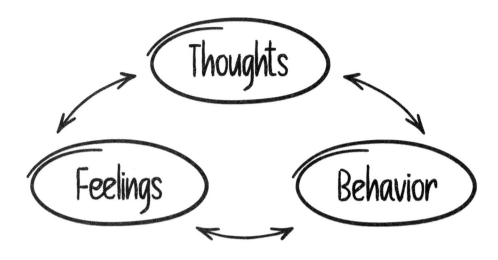

Figure 4.3 Cognitive Triangle

Recall that we divided the flavors of fear into these same three categories. Consider how a fearful thought (*Uh oh, if I get a headache today, then I won't be able to meet my work deadline!*) could cause you to experience a fearful feeling (anxiety), which could cause you to engage in a fearful behavior (repeatedly checking on the sensations in your head to make sure you don't have a headache). And before you know it, the pain–fear cycle is off and running with a chain reaction of fearful thoughts, feelings, and behaviors that cause pain. This is one not-so-fun example of how thoughts, feelings, and behaviors are interconnected.

The good news is that we can also use the way that thoughts, feelings, and behaviors are interconnected to our advantage. Again, if fear is the fuel that keeps pain burning, a sense of safety is the fire extinguisher that puts out the flames. By learning how to think, feel, and behave in ways that ground our nervous systems in a sense of safety, we interrupt the pain–fear cycle's momentum, gradually slowing it down until it eventually stops spinning.

Thoughts

The exercises in this section focus on harnessing the power of thoughts. Whereas certain types of thoughts are fuel for the pain–fear cycle, these exercises will explore how other types of thoughts can have the opposite effect. Harnessing the power of thoughts might initially feel awkward or even inauthentic, but stick with it and keep practicing. The more your nervous system gets the hang of this new way of thinking, the more comfortable it will become.

EXERCISE: Engaging with Recovery Stories

One powerful way to strengthen your foundation of safety is also one of the easiest. When you engage with other peoples' stories of recovery from chronic pain, you help your brain connect with its own potential to heal.

Some of our favorite recovery story resources are listed in the additional resources section at the end of this book. Choose three of those recovery stories to engage with—for example, watch a film, listen to a podcast episode, and read a recovery forum post. After engaging with each recovery story, take a few minutes to reflect on your response to it.

Recovery Story	Your Reflections

Feel free to engage with more recovery stories if you like. Each time you connect to a recovery story in a positive way, you add another brick to your foundation of safety.

Many practices that harness the power of thoughts involve *self-talk*, which is just a fancy name for thoughts you direct toward yourself. Everyone regularly engages in self-talk, but most of it is by default. What we're offering here is intentional self-talk: thoughts that you consciously choose to direct toward yourself with a particular goal in mind.

EXERCISE: Practicing Your Self-Talk Tone

If the goal of intentional self-talk is to soothe your nervous system—to impart a sense of safety— tone is important. This exercise is aimed at helping you zero in on the soothing tone you will use when engaging in self-talk practices.

Imagine that you're taking care of a young child you care for very much. They wake up in the middle of the night terrified, convinced there are monsters under the bed. They come to you seeking safety and comfort.

You empathize with the child's very real fear, but you also know the fear is a false alarm—there are no monsters under the bed, and the child is perfectly safe. Imagine soothing the child, giving them permission not to worry. Imagine the soft, warm, reassuring tone you would use. Practice using this tone aloud, saying "You're safe now. Nothing is going to hurt you."

Practice saying these phrases aloud a few times, getting a feel for the soothing tone you would use. Notice how it feels in your body to speak with this calm, caring, and confident voice. If other messages arise that you'd like to share with this imaginary child, go ahead and say those with the same soothing tone.

Use this same tone of voice whenever you're engaging in soothing self-talk practices, whether you are vocalizing the self-talk aloud or silently to yourself. Any time you have trouble finding the tone in the future, return to this exercise to help you remember.

★ EXERCISE: Reflecting on the Evidence

Return to the self-assessment exercise in chapter 2 and review all the signs of neuroplastic pain that resonated with your own experience. List below the signs that resonated most. If there are other things you've learned in this workbook or elsewhere that support the notion that you experience neuroplastic pain, list those here as well.

Evidence That Your Pain Is Neuroplastic

_____

_____

_____

_____

_____

_____

_____

_____

When you notice your mind spinning about what illness you might have or what serious medical treatment you might need, reflect on these pieces of evidence as well as everything you've learned about how neuroplastic pain works. Using a warm, reassuring tone, remind yourself that being in pain is not the same as being in danger.

EXERCISE: Self-Talk Script

Each of us has a few flavors of fear that we know particularly well—the worries that we've encountered a thousand times over, the frustrations we've struggled with for as long as we can remember, the old habit of numbing ourself to avoid the pain. These familiar neural pathways can feel like they have a gravitational force of their own, pulling us back down them again and again, even when we know that they won't lead us anywhere we want to go.

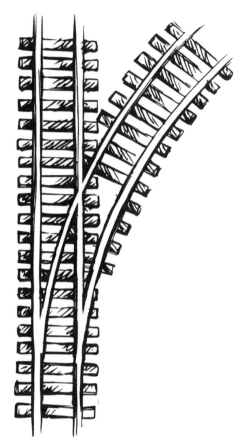

A well-worn neural pathway is like a train track. Once your brain is barreling down it, it can feel nearly impossible to change directions. But with the right tricks, changing directions is possible. By intentionally laying another track right next to the one you want to leave behind, you give your brain somewhere else to go.

The secret lies in making sure the new track is big and sturdy enough to give your brain—which is barreling down the old track with all the momentum of a high-speed loco-motive—something it can firmly switch onto. The self-talk script in this exercise will help. By the time you're done reading it, your brain will be miles away from the old neural pathway you left behind.

Using a soothing, reassuring tone, slowly read the fol-lowing script to yourself, making sure to really think through each line before moving onto the next.

Figure 4.4
Learning to Switch Tracks

Line 1	*Hello, brain. I know you're afraid.*
Line 2	*This pain is caused by learned neural pathways, not real danger.*
Line 3	*You learned to err on the side of caution because you wanted to keep me safe.*
Line 4	*I appreciate you for all you've done to protect me, but now it's okay to relax.*
Line 5	*Together we can learn a new and safer way of being.*

Once you've read through the whole script, go ahead and rewrite it below to help you remember it. You can rewrite it, word for word, or you can play around with changing the language to sound more like you. If your flavor of fear is anger, frustration, or another emotion altogether, you can replace "afraid" in line 1 with whatever emotion resonates most. If you experience other neuroplastic symptoms, you can switch out the word "pain" for "itchiness," "dizziness," "fatigue," or other symptoms. You can also try replacing the word "brain" in the first line with the name that you gave your protective part when you were getting to know your inner protectors in chapter 3. You can swap out the pronouns, from "you" to "I" to "we," and use whichever feels best. Keep tweaking the language until you land on words that feel true to you.

Line 1	
Line 2	
Line 3	
Line 4	
Line 5	

Now that you've written your own self-talk script, it's time to put it into practice. Take a photo of the script on your smartphone, or write it on an index card that you keep in your wallet. When you notice pain—and especially when you notice flavors of fear surrounding the pain—slowly read through this script from top to bottom aloud or silently, making sure to use the same soothing, reassuring self-talk tone that you practiced earlier. As you read the script to yourself, you may also try placing a hand on your heart to amplify your sense of comfort and safety.

If you experience pain during much of the day, every day, aim to practice this script at least three times a day for two weeks. If your pain is more intermittent, simply practice the self-talk script when you notice that pain has arisen. Each time you practice responding to pain by practicing this script, you're inviting your brain to switch tracks from an old neural pathway that perpetuates the pain–fear cycle to a new neural pathway that builds your foundation of safety.

At the end of your first two weeks of practice, or whenever you feel it's appropriate, come back to this workbook to journal about your experience using the script. Did it help? What challenges did you experience? What else did you notice?

_____

_____

_____

_____

_____

★ EXERCISE: Self-Talk Minis

Once you've practiced the full self-talk script several times and feel comfortable with it, you can begin to use shorter self-talk phrases. We call these shorter phrases *self-talk minis*.

Use these minis when you want to give your brain a little reminder but don't feel like you need your full self-talk script. Maybe you're feeling just a twinge of pain rather than an intense sensation, or perhaps you notice yourself starting to tense up in response to a trigger, but the flavors of fear haven't really set in yet. Experiment with trying out the different self-talk minis listed here, and feel free to create your own in the blank spaces provided. Practice your favorites regularly as needed. Whether you say these self-talk minis aloud or silently, remember to use the warm and reassuring tone that you've been practicing.

Self-Talk Minis
It's okay.
I know you're scared—I'm here with you.
Hello brain, I know you're trying to protect me, and I appreciate you for that.
The pain switch is stuck in the on position, and even though it hurts, I'm okay.

I know it hurts, but you're safe.
This pain is caused by learned neural pathways, not real danger.
Thank you for trying to protect me, but I'm safe now—it's okay to relax.
It hurts right now, but it's only temporary.
My body is healthy and strong.

Feelings

This section is about helping you feel safe. What does it mean to feel safe? It's different for different people, and there's no one answer that feels true to everyone. In general, when we talk about feeling safe, we are talking about a feeling that is the opposite of high alert. Many people describe this feeling as grounded, relaxed, or calm.

While we're on board with the idea that you can't change the way you're already feeling in this very moment, there are actually a whole lot of things you can do to change the way you feel in the next moment and all the moments after that. It's a matter of self-regulation: learning the way your body functions and how to work with it so you can stay calm and respond to your experience, rather than being overwhelmed by it.

In neuroscience-speak, we say that you feel safe when your *parasympathetic nervous system* is activated. The parasympathetic nervous system is the part of your nervous system that helps your body relax—including after the experience of stress. It also helps run some of the most essential body functions, like digestion, immune response, sexual arousal, and mood. This is in contrast to the *sympathetic nervous system*, which is the part of your nervous system that activates in a *fight-or-flight* response: your heart races, your breathing becomes shallow, your muscles tense, and you feel anything but safe. And as you already know, the more unsafe you feel, the faster the pain–fear cycle spins.

Luckily, we all have a reset switch running through our bodies that helps our brains transition from danger mode to safety mode. This reset switch is called the *vagus nerve*, and it's a communication superhighway that connects your brain with all of your essential organs.

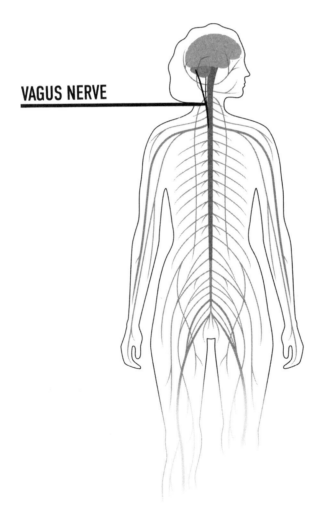

VAGUS NERVE

Figure 4.5 Vagus Nerve

When the vagus nerve is stimulated, your heart rate slows, sending the signal to the rest of your body that danger has passed and it's time to relax. As a result, your body feels safe, which interrupts the pain–fear cycle and strengthens your foundation of safety. There are many ways to stimulate the vagus nerve, and we focus here on two of our favorites. We encourage you to build these practices into your daily life on a regular and ongoing basis.

★ EXERCISE: Cold Pack Relaxation

About a year into the coronavirus pandemic—and the tidal wave of the anxiety that came with it—a strange new health trend began sweeping the internet. While we don't think that all internet health trends are worthy of your attention, this approach to vagus nerve stimulation offers one of the most easily accessible ways to soothe the nervous system. Our favorite option is a reusable gel ice pack, but you can use a bag of frozen peas or corn if that's what you have on hand. Note: If you're hesitant to try this exercise for any reason, which may include traumatic associations with feelings of cold, please feel free to skip this exercise and move ahead.

Remove your cold pack from the freezer and wrap it with cloth to protect your skin. Recline or lie down, so your back is fully supported, and place the wrapped cold pack against the center of your upper chest, with your hands crossed over the cold pack, gently pressing the cold pack onto your chest. You should be able to feel a strong sensation of coldness on your chest, but not so cold that it hurts or irritates your skin. Adjust the cloth as needed to find the right balance. Plan to stay in this position, continuing to hold the cold pack against your chest for at least ten minutes. If you're comfortable closing your eyes, please do.

Now imagine that the cold pack is a powerful magnet for your attention, sucking all your awareness into the feeling of coldness in your chest. With each inhale, breathe more of your awareness into that intense sensation of coldness, then hold your breath there for a moment before relaxing into a long, slow exhale. Continue like this for some time. As your awareness continues to gravitate toward the cold, notice what happens to your emotions. If at any point you notice your attention drifting toward thoughts or other sensations in the body, that's no problem—just use an inhalation to gently invite your awareness back into the feeling of coldness in your chest.

Once ten minutes have passed, but before you change positions or remove the cold pack, check back in with the rest of your body. What do you notice? Are things different in any way than when you began? Has the pace or content of your thinking changed? What words would you use to describe your emotional state?

For many people, cold pack relaxation is a powerful way to acquaint the nervous system with feelings of calm and safety. When you are first starting out, aim to practice this once a day for two weeks. You can also use this exercise as needed when feelings of pain or distress arise. After engaging regularly for two weeks, feel free to be more flexible with both timing and frequency. Remember that this tool is here for you any time your nervous system could use some soothing.

Learning to Breathe

Imagine your long-ago ancestor, running as fast as she could from a lion on the savanna. This was the kind of danger that our bodies were built to protect us from: physical threats to our safety that we needed to run away from or fight against. As a result, when our brains perceive danger, our breathing becomes quick and shallow, our muscles tense, and we are pumped full of adrenaline, ready to respond with fight or with flight as needed.

Most of the threats we experience in modern life aren't threats to our physical safety but are financial, emotional, political, professional, logistical, and interpersonal. Still, the part of your brain that responds to danger can't tell the difference between physical threats like the lion and psychological threats like the ones we more commonly face today. When the brain perceives danger—no matter what kind—it automatically responds with quick, shallow breathing and tense muscles. For this reason, many of us navigating the everyday stresses of modern life exist in a near constant state of agitation. Add chronic pain to the equation, and feelings of safety become even harder to access.

Luckily, we can reverse engineer this process. By intentionally breathing slowly and deeply, we stimulate the vagus nerve, sending the message to the whole body that the danger has passed and it's safe to relax. For many of us, this will take practice. Especially if we've spent much of our lives breathing quick shallow breaths, learning to breathe deeply can take some time, but it's worth the effort. Because you breathe all day every day, how you breathe has a big impact on how you feel and is one of the most powerful ways to build your foundation of safety.

★ **EXERCISE:** Deep Belly Breathing

When just starting out, many people find deep belly breathing more accessible lying down. If you're able to lie down comfortably, please do so. Feel free to prop up your knees or legs if you like. If you prefer sitting, position yourself so that your back feels fully supported.

Once you are in a relaxed and comfortable position, place your left hand over the center of your chest and your right hand just above your belly button and a few inches to the right. Close your eyes and, without thinking too much about it, take a deep breath in through your nose and out through your mouth. Notice which hand moved more—was it your right hand or your left hand?

Now, keeping your eyes closed, once again inhale deeply through your nose. Breathe the air deep into your belly—imagine bringing the air all the way below your belly button—and then exhale slowly through your mouth. Notice again, which hand moved more?

Continue to inhale through your nose and exhale through your mouth, gently inviting the air more deeply into your belly. At the end of the inhale, try holding your breath in your belly for a count of three, then exhale slowly through your mouth for a count of four.

See if, using only your breath, you can make your right hand move more than your left hand. You may explore applying some gentle pressure to your chest with your left hand to remind your body that you are breathing into your belly, not your chest. Keep going like this for about ten minutes.

If you find this exercise difficult or frustrating, don't be discouraged. Your muscles, lungs, and nervous system have been breathing another way for a very long time. Trust that, as you continue to practice in the days and weeks ahead, deep belly breathing will start to come more naturally.

When starting out, we suggest setting aside at least ten minutes a day for deep belly breathing. You may find it easiest to practice for ten minutes after you wake up or ten minutes before sleep. As you begin to become more comfortable with deep belly breathing, you are welcome to combine it with cold pack relaxation.

The more you practice, the more you will find it possible to take deep breaths throughout your day, not just during designated periods of deep belly breathing. Eventually, you may find that deep, slow breathing is even occurring on its own. If you notice that happening, take a moment to check in with your body and celebrate. Recognize that changing old habits is hard work, and this change happened because of choices that you made.

Leaning into Pleasure

For most people experiencing chronic pain, pain intensity ebbs and flows. And many find that periods of decreased pain often coincide with doing something pleasurable, like sitting in the sunshine on a nice day, snuggling a pet, or eating a delicious meal. One reason for this is fairly obvious: when pain is less intense, you're more able to fully engage with the activities you enjoy and to fully recognize them as enjoyable. But another reason is just as important: feelings of pleasure ground the nervous system in a sense of safety. Much like stimulating the vagus nerve, leaning into pleasure is a way of switching from danger mode to safety mode.

★ EXERCISE: Leaning into Pleasant Sensation[2]

Leaning into a sensation is something we do with our bodies. We allow our sense of touch to gravitate into and fully inhabit the sensation.

To start out, position yourself as comfortably as possible. This can be sitting, lying down, standing, walking—whatever position feels best. You may find it helpful to close your eyes.

Allow your awareness to gravitate into a part of your body that doesn't hurt. Try the palms of your hands or the soles of your feet. Alternatively, you can use the sensation of your breath coming in and out of your belly or nostrils. Whatever you choose, allow your awareness to completely gravitate into the sensations in that part of your body. Allow yourself to really feel into it, even if only for a moment or two at a time.

Sinking your sense of touch more fully into the sensation, is there any part of this experience that is pleasurable? Maybe you feel a subtle tingling on your palms or in the soles of your feet. If you're using breathing, notice the sensation of your belly completely filling with air...Then hold your breath for a count of three, and allow yourself to enjoy the feeling of release on the exhale.

We aren't looking for fireworks here—just some part of your body that feels even just a tiny bit nice. Allow your awareness to fully inhabit that part of your body. Live there. Lean into it. Stay with the sensation, and see if you can allow yourself to enjoy it just a little bit more.

2   Note that this tool is often referred to as leaning into *positive* sensation (Gordon and Ziv 2021).

Practice leaning into pleasant sensation to soothe your nervous system when you are feeling pain or distress. You can also practice it when you're not in pain, which will strengthen your brain's foundation of safety. The more you practice leaning into pleasant sensation, the easier it will become. As pleasant sensations become more accessible, you may find that you no longer need to get into a comfortable position or close your eyes to connect with them.

In addition to leaning into pleasant sensations that are already in your body, you can intentionally bring about pleasant experiences, giving yourself something enjoyable to lean into.

★ EXERCISE: Conjuring Pleasant Experience

Review the list below, putting a check mark next to the experiences you'd be willing to try, and adding any of your own ideas at the end.

Pleasant Experiences

Give yourself a hand massage with your favorite hand lotion.

Light your favorite incense or a scented candle or apply your favorite essential oil.

Take a hot bath or shower.

Run your hands under warm water.

Snuggle with your pet.

Drink a warm cup of tea.

Listen to a song that makes you feel good.

Stimulate your scalp with your fingertips or a head massager.

Masturbate.

Savor a delicious snack.

Fill a hot water bottle and put it on whatever part of your body feels best.

Get cozy with a soft blanket or a stuffed animal.

Lie down under the blankets and rub your bare feet against each other.

Engage with some gentle stretching.

_____

_____

_____

_____

_____

Choose one or more of these pleasant experiences to explore. Practice intentionally leaning into just how pleasant the experience really is. Allow your felt awareness to gravitate around your sense of touch, taste, smell, or hearing, and completely sink into that feeling of enjoyment.

When you find yourself in the midst of everyday pleasant experiences—the smell of your morning coffee, the taste of a yummy meal, the feeling of lying down for the first time after a long day—take a few moments to lean into that experience and enjoy just how pleasurable it can be. Every time you connect with pleasure in this way, you add another brick to your foundation of safety.

Behaviors

As we've discussed, many behaviors can perpetuate the pain–fear cycle. In chapter 2, you spent some time looking at how certain behaviors as they arise in your own lived experience can contribute to your pain. Awareness and understanding is the first step.

The next step is to intentionally practice new ways of behaving, establishing new neural pathways so that your old behavioral habits don't have the same pull they once did. The exercises in this section will help you explore new and safer ways of behaving toward yourself and the world around you.

EXERCISE: Connecting with Kindness

You may notice a common theme in this book: we're encouraging you again and again, in different ways, to practice being kind toward yourself. While our habitual pattern may be to relate to parts of ourselves that we don't like with fear, judgment, anger, avoidance, or control, each of us also contains the natural capacity to relate to those same parts with compassion. The goal of this exercise is to help you connect with this natural capacity for kindness in greater depth.

Take a moment to imagine that you are shopping in a crowded department store on a busy weekend afternoon. You are about to visit one last shop before heading home when you notice a small child standing by himself, looking lost. He begins to cry, and you realize it's up to you to help him.

Upon realizing that the child is lost and scared, what emotions do you feel toward him? Where do you feel those emotions in your body?

_____

_____

_____

_____

_____

How do you approach the child? What is your body posture like? What are your facial expressions?

_____

_____

_____

_____

_____

When you begin to speak to him, how would you describe your tone of voice? Do you speak slowly or quickly? Softly or loudly? What message are you trying to communicate through the way that you speak to him?

_____

_____

_____

_____

What words do you say? What questions do you ask?

_____

_____

_____

_____

How are you trying to help him feel? To that end, what are some things you are careful not to do?

_____

_____

_____

_____

There is no one right answer to these questions. Rather, this exercise is about tapping into your natural capacity to befriend and support. Take a moment to acknowledge that this capacity for kindness is already within you.

Learning to behave toward yourself in the same way that you would behave toward an imaginary child may not come easily at first. But learning to direct that same kindness toward yourself is just a matter of practice.

When you notice that you are relating to pain—or other aspects of your inner experience—with fear, judgment, anger, avoidance, or control, take a moment to pause. Take a deep breath, acknowledging the old habit and inviting it to step back. Then imagine back to the lost child in the department store, connecting with the ways you would behave toward him. Then try relating to your own experience from that same place.

Each time you practice behaving toward yourself in this way, even if only for a moment or two, you strengthen these new neural pathways, further strengthening your foundation of safety.

Rewiring your brain can be hard work. But, believe it or not, developing new neural pathways can also be fun. We swear it. The final two exercises in this chapter invite you to play around with old behaviors in new ways.

Two of the most common patterns of behavior that we see in people struggling with chronic pain are preoccupation and intensity. When left unchecked, each of these behavior patterns, in its own way, fuels the pain–fear cycle. As you begin to see these old behavior patterns clearly and choose to relate to them with a lighthearted attitude—and maybe even a sense of humor—you end up accomplishing two things. First, you bring awareness to the old habit so it no longer has the same hold that it did when you were unknowingly caught in its grip. Second, by practicing new behaviors in a playful and lighthearted way, you teach the brain that this new way of doing things is actually kind of fun—and as we already learned, enjoying yourself is one great way to strengthen your safety network.

Playing with Preoccupation

Preoccupation is the tendency to fixate on one particular thing. In the world of chronic pain, preoccupation with physical symptoms is understandable. When pain is constantly getting in the way of the life you want to be living, it's only natural to focus on it and to do everything you can to stop it. The problem is that preoccupation with the pain and how it's affecting our lives gives rise to more fearful thoughts and feelings, fueling the very pain that we so desperately want to go away.

So, what can you do about preoccupation? One of the best ways to break the habit is to proactively give your brain something else to engage with. You get extra points if that something else is at least a little bit fun, because the more fun an activity is, the more engrossing it will be.

The following challenges give your preoccupied brain something else to chew on. Give one of these a try when you notice that your brain is fixating on your pain or how it's affecting you and you want to help it switch tracks. If along the way you notice that your brain wants to return to its old habit of preoccupation, just gently invite your attention back to the challenge at hand and keep going.

Count colors: Look around you. From your current vantage point, how many things can you see right now that are red? Count them, making sure not to miss a single one. Now, how many things can you see that are orange? Okay, count those. How about yellow? Green? See if you can make it all the way through your old buddy ROY G. BIV, counting the colors as you go.

Listen up: Open up your ears, identifying as many distinct sounds as you can for a full three minutes. This challenge is especially fun outside, but it can work indoors too. If you're with someone else, you can turn listening up into a friendly competition. Trading off, see how many sounds each of you can find. Keep going until there are no more distinct sounds in your awareness.

Sing along: Choose a song that you love but don't already know all the words to. Look up the lyrics online and try singing along to the whole song, every word, note for note. The idea isn't to get it perfect. It's to allow your attention to get totally absorbed in the challenge of singing the song from beginning to end and have fun along the way.

Boogie on: Is there a dance move you've always wanted to learn? Look up a tutorial online and learn how to do it. If you're not sure where to start, search "beginner line dance tutorial" and see what you find. If you have limited mobility, try searching "hand jive tutorial" and give that a try. Again, this isn't about doing the moves perfectly—it's about giving your brain something different to chew on.

Puzzle me this: Sudoku, Wordle, crosswords, and other puzzles are fantastic ways to break a pattern of preoccupation. The trick is finding the right balance so that the puzzle is challenging enough to keep your attention but not so challenging that you become frustrated.

One of our favorite ways to employ these brain games is as a means of interrupting the old neural pathways that we identified in the "Pain Maps" exercise in chapter 3. Take the example that Olivia gave for that exercise: getting a headache every time she engaged in aerobic activity. Through PRT, Olivia learned that it is not her elevated heart rate that gives her headaches but rather the many flavors of fear that arise in response to it. While the intellectual part of Olivia now understands that the pulsing at her temples doesn't have to be the first sign that a headache is coming on, it's how she responds to the pulsing at her temples that matters. She knows that if she fixates on the pulsing, she will probably get a headache, just as she feared. So, instead, she uses a brain game to shift her attention somewhere else. She opens up her ears, and one by one, starts picking out every single sound that she can for a full three minutes. If she notices her attention being pulled toward the pulsing at her temples, she gently brings it back to the sounds around her—a bird singing, the wind in the trees, a car starting up down the block. Gradually, by practicing this over and over when she's out running, she breaks the pattern of preoccupation that has kept her locked in the pain–fear cycle for so long.

Decreasing Intensity

Doing things with intensity can be a really good thing. When we do things with intensity, we give 110 percent. We go hard. We pull out all the stops. We really go for it. Does this sound like you? If so, your capacity to do things this way has almost certainly helped you in too many ways to count.

The problem is that doing things with intensity can also have a downside, especially when it becomes habitual. When we do things with intensity, we are often, well…*tense*—both emotionally and physically. In fact, the word "intense" comes from a Latin word meaning "stretched tightly" or "strained."

You learned earlier in this chapter about how you can help your brain switch from danger mode (the sympathetic nervous system) to safety mode (the parasympathetic nervous system). Breathing deeply signals to your nervous system that all is well, causing your brain to switch into safety mode. On the other hand, behaving as if you're in danger—that is, doing things in a tense, quick, or pressured way—can reinforce the nervous system's sense that it's in danger, causing the brain to double down on danger mode.

Say you're cleaning the bathroom with intensity. You may think you're just doing a really excellent job! But the part of your brain that responds to threat comes to believe, consciously or not, that your life depends on it. In this way, doing things with intensity—powering through each step in a hurry to get to the next—causes the pain–fear cycle to spin on in the same way that flavors of fear do. By contrast, learning to do things in a relaxed and low-stakes manner sends the message to the brain that all is well, strengthening the underlying foundation of safety.

EXERCISE: Playing with Intensity

One powerful way of decreasing intensity is learning to slow down. This exercise is about doing just that.

Take out your smartphone and open your favorite social media app. If you don't have social media, your favorite news media website or blog will work as well.

Take a moment and just start scrolling as you normally would. Zip on by each post. Notice this, notice that. Like this post. Comment on that one. Share one with a friend. Skim the content as you go, however you would typically engage. Keep on going in this manner for a few minutes.

Speeding through social media in this way might not feel intense to you. In fact, it might even feel comfortable, a familiar way of relaxing when you have a few free minutes. However, speeding through things in this way—hurrying through one moment just to make it to the next—is a hallmark of intensity. Remember that something can feel comfortable because it's familiar, but comfort doesn't necessarily translate into a sense of safety for your nervous system.

Okay, now return to the top. Scroll through the same material you just did, but see if you can scroll more slowly than you did before. As you scroll, pause to notice what you see. Label the colors you see on the page: *pink, blue, purple.* Label some of the objects you see in the images you are scrolling by: *puppy, smiles, sandwich.* Take a moment to breathe deeply before scrolling from one post to the next.

As you continue to scroll, see if you can pick up on details that you didn't notice before. Go slowly enough to label what you see in the background: *tree, pickup truck, sand.* Read the full names of the people posting. Read through the captions and comments, and take the time to identify how they make you feel: *amused, angry, awkward.*

As you scroll in this slower, more observant way, notice how it feels in your body. What is your breathing like? What's happening with your shoulders? How about your jaw? Observe whether there is a change and, if so, what that change feels like.

Going forward, when you notice that you're doing something with intensity—operating at full throttle, or hurrying through from one moment to the next—take a moment to pause. Remember how it felt to scroll in a slow, observant, low-stakes way, and invite that same slow and easeful energy into whatever you're doing.

Learning the Steps

In this chapter, you've harnessed the power of thoughts, feelings, and behaviors to strengthen your foundation of safety. As you reprocess pain in the chapters to come, you'll deepen your acquaintance with the way that both danger and safety *feel* in your body. Then you may wish to revisit this chapter in its entirety to use your newfound awareness to strengthen your foundation of safety even further. Notice that the healing process described here is not linear. In PRT, you don't recover from chronic pain by completing one step, once and for all, before moving on to the next. Rather, the healing process is more like a dance: you shift your weight from strengthening your foundation of safety to rewiring pain pathways, and then from rewiring pain pathways back to strengthening your foundation...and so on. The more you familiarize yourself with these steps, the more momentum they'll have. And before you know it, you'll be gliding across the dance floor of your recovery as effortlessly as Gene Kelly tapping his way down that rainy sidewalk.

CHAPTER 5

Rewiring Your Pain Pathways

Your brain sure has come a long way since you started this workbook. First, you learned what neuroplastic pain is, how it works, and the crucial role that fear plays in perpetuating pain. Then, you began to befriend your own nervous system, becoming aware of the way that the pain–fear cycle operates in your own mind and body. Finally, you started taking steps to strengthen new neural pathways that help to build your brain's foundation of safety.

All this hard work has helped prepare your nervous system for the main event: learning to relate to your own pain in a new way. As you've come to understand, fear primes the brain to perceive sensation through a lens of danger, making the brain far more likely to mistake neutral sensations for dangerous ones, and send a pain signal in response. However, when the brain perceives that same neutral sensation through a lens of safety, it will be able to see that sensation for what it really is: totally harmless. The more adept the brain becomes at perceiving sensation through a lens of safety, the more accurately it will distinguish between harmless and dangerous sensations, and the less neuroplastic pain you will feel. This chapter is focused on helping your brain learn how to do this.

Exploring Sensation Through a Lens of Safety

Recall the example of the bear and the stump from chapter 2. Having heard about a bear attack nearby, you're walking through the forest and see a bear in the distance. However, it's actually not a bear at all—it's just a big old stump. Your brain, understandably on "high alert" due to the news of the recent attack, perceived the shadowy figure through a lens of danger, mistaking the stump for a bear.

So far in this workbook, our focus has been on understanding why your brain would make this kind of mistake. You have learned about how fear distorts perception and why some nervous systems are more prone to fear than others. But in this chapter, we want to shift the focus to a new question: Once your brain has made this mistake, what can you do to correct it?

To answer this question, let's return to the forest. Imagine you're standing there by yourself, still seeing what you believe to be a bear in the distance. Your adrenaline is pumping and your survival instinct is screaming at you to run in the other direction. Just as you turn back toward the campground to run to safety, you see another camper coming your way. "Turn around!" you shout at the top of your lungs, pointing at the shadowy figure in the distance. "There's a huge bear!"

But the other camper never heard about the recent bear attack, so she's strolling through the forest on this beautiful day, just as calm as can be. She looks where you're pointing, doing her best to figure out what you're shouting about. "I'm sorry," she says to you calmly. "But I don't see any bears out there. All I see is a big old stump."

You're in complete disbelief. *How can she not see that humongous bear?* Your initial instinct is still to run, but you don't feel right leaving this hapless camper all by herself… and well, she does seem fairly certain there's no bear. And also, you have to admit, you do feel a lot safer now that someone is with you. With your nervous system calmed and your curiosity ignited, you decide to give it one more look. You peer back in the direction of the bear and…lo and behold…*the other camper was right*. Where you once saw fur, you now see brown bark and fuzzy moss. Where you once saw legs, you now see thick roots. And where you once saw the bear's massive head, you now see nothing but a big knotty burl. The bear you were sure you saw really is just a harmless stump.

Two things helped here: one, by engaging your foundation of safety, the lens of danger dropped away; and two, viewing the shadowy figure with genuine curiosity enabled you to see it for what it really was.

While the example of the bear and the stump is about your sense of sight, your other senses work the same way. If you view sensory input through a lens of danger, you will be more likely to mistake something harmless for something dangerous. By interrupting the fear cycle and adding some curiosity to the mix, you will be able to perceive what's out there for what it really is. Similarly, in the realm of chronic pain, learning to investigate bodily sensations through a lens of safety will allow you to *feel* those sensations for what they really are.

EXERCISE: Let Your Sense of Touch Do the Thinking

While we might assume that when we see, touch, or hear something, we're perceiving that thing as it really is, neuroscience research suggests this is not the case. Rather, according to the theory known as *predictive coding*, the brain is constantly forming a model of its surroundings and using that model to predict sensory inputs. The theory states that our sensory perceptions are, at least in part, determined by those predictions. Predictive coding helps explain why stories like the bear and the stump are not so uncommon in the real world.

As a result of this natural predictive tendency, learning to feel things as they really are—rather than as our brains predict them to be—can take some practice. This exercise is intended to help you strengthen your capacity to passively receive sensory input rather than allow the prediction machine in your head to run the show. Learning to do this now will really come in handy later on.

Wherever you are right now, take out your hand and prepare to touch some stuff. Choose an object within reach and rub your fingertips against it—how does the object feel? Your brain may come up with some answers before you've even really made contact with the object—the desk is obviously hard, right? Well, try to put those predictions aside for now, and slow down enough to let your sense of touch do the thinking. Allow your fingertips to answer the question for you: How does the desk really feel?

It may be helpful to close your eyes. Take your time to come up with at least three texture or sensation words to describe what you're touching. Be careful that the words you're choosing are words that describe your sense of touch. For example, if you find yourself describing something as "plastic" or "metal," notice that these are mental concepts that describe what you're touching, not how it feels. If your instinct is to describe something as "shiny," that word describes visual perception rather than touch. You may find it helpful to imagine that you don't know what object you're touching and all you have is your sense of touch to guide you. Allow your hands to continue exploring until your sense of touch finds a sensation word to describe the object (like "hard," "smooth," or "cool").

If you need some help finding the right words to describe what you're feeling, check out the list of sensation words that follows this exercise. Once your sense of touch has landed on three sensation words to describe how the first object feels, move on to another object. Continue on with this process of exploration for at least five different objects.

Object	Sensation 1	Sensation 2	Sensation 3

Although your brain will get the hang of it eventually, finding the right words to describe your felt experience can be a little tricky at first. When you're not quite sure how to describe something, you can refer to this list to find the right words to describe the physical sensation you're feeling at this moment.

The Big List of Sensation Words

hard	soft	warm	cool
rough	smooth	sharp	dull
tight	loose	bumpy	level
fuzzy	prickly	heavy	light
empty	full	tingling	numb
dense	spacious	burning	icy
sticky	slippery	wet	dry
pulsing	vibrating	twitching	throbbing
undulating	tingling	expanding	contracting

Untangling Sensation and Fear

Sensory perception—in the case of the sense of touch, what something *feels* like—is not simply a reflection of the way things actually are. Rather, our sensory perception is influenced by a whole variety of factors. Flavors of fear, in particular, can be especially powerful in this regard, causing otherwise neutral sensations to feel mightily unpleasant. Rewiring your pain pathways is, in large part, a matter of untangling sensation from the fearful beliefs and emotions that we have surrounding that sensation.

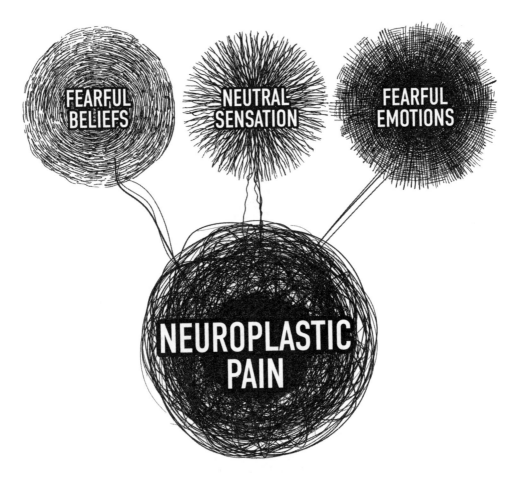

Figure 5.1 Untangling Sensation from Fear

To better understand the concept of untangling a sensation from the fear surrounding it, take this example: Imagine dipping your foot into a steaming hot bath at the end of a long hard day. The sensation is intensely hot, but it's also very welcome. As you dip your foot deeper under the surface, gradually adjusting to the temperature of the tub, the intense heat feels deeply pleasurable.

Now, imagine a completely different scene: waking up in the middle of the night because your foot is boiling hot. This has been happening every night for months, and your doctors can't figure out what's going on or what to do about it. You're completely exhausted, and all you want to do is sleep, but the sensation of intense heat in your foot won't go away, no matter what you do. You're in tremendous discomfort, and your distress is understandable.

In both of these scenarios, the raw physical sensation is the same. But the intense heat is deeply pleasurable in one instance and profoundly unpleasant in the other. Whether that same raw sensation feels pleasant or unpleasant depends on your beliefs and emotions around it. In the case of the bath, you *welcome* the heat and understand why it's happening—you experience neither an ounce of distress around the sensation nor resistance to it. As a result, your brain is able to perceive the sensation through a lens of safety, and the intense heat isn't just neutral—it's downright pleasant. On the other hand, in the case of waking up in the middle of the night, you have no clue where the sensation is coming from, and it's gotten in the way of your much-needed sleep night after night. You feel substantial distress around the situation, causing your brain to perceive the sensation through a lens of danger. As a result, the intense heat you feel is profoundly unpleasant.

Although the raw sensation is the same in both cases, it's the absence of fearful beliefs and emotions in the first instance and the presence of them in the other that cause you to have such vastly different physical experiences. If you were able to untangle those fearful beliefs and emotions from the sensation, then your foot in bed would not actually feel so different from your foot in the tub.

Much of this workbook so far has focused on untangling sensation from the fearful beliefs you may have around it—helping your brain to understand that pain does not necessarily mean danger. The next exercise will help you begin to untangle sensation from the fearful emotions surrounding it to allow your brain to perceive the underlying sensation more clearly.

★ EXERCISE: Scaling Unpleasantness and Distress

Once you understand the way that emotional distress can become tangled up with sensations to make them more, well, distressing, what are you supposed to do about it? In our experience, this level of understanding is usually necessary for healing but not sufficient. To move toward recovery, you will need to transform your intellectual understanding into lived experience.

This exercise offers a simple but powerful way to help your brain distinguish between a physical sensation and the emotions you have about that sensation. This exercise is designed for moments when you are experiencing physical symptoms. If you're not experiencing any physical symptoms right now, then set the workbook aside and return to this exercise the next time your physical symptoms arise.

Check in with the physical discomfort you're experiencing at this very moment. Find where in your body the sensation is most intense. On a scale of 0 to 10, how unpleasant is this sensation? Circle the intensity of your sensation on this scale:

0   1   2   3   4   5   6   7   8   9   10

not unpleasant at all   most unpleasant imaginable

Now, check in with the distress you're feeling about that sensation, or the resistance you're feeling to it. Where in your body do you feel that distress or resistance? On the following scale of 0 to 10, how much distress or resistance are you experiencing? Circle the level of intensity. (Note that we use "distress" and "resistance" throughout this chapter, but if those words don't resonate for you, that's okay—what we're trying to get in touch with is any aversive emotion that you might be feeling in this moment. For support, refer to the middle column in the "Flavors of Fear" exercise in chapter 2, and feel free to use whatever word is the best fit for you.)

0   1   2   3   4   5   6   7   8   9   10

no distress/resistance   most distress/resistance imaginable

Once you've checked in with your level of distress, go back and check in with unpleasantness again. What do you notice? There is no right or wrong answer here. And we don't expect this exercise to be a magic wand that makes your neuroplastic pain disappear in an instant. The goal is simply to train your brain to perceive sensation and emotion surrounding the sensation as two distinct experiences. As long as you're able to connect with each of these experiences separately—even if you feel them in the same part of your body or if the number for one happens to be the same as the number for the other—you're doing your job perfectly.

Get in the habit of scaling both unpleasantness of the sensation and distress about the sensation regularly. Perhaps do this once daily if you're in pain every day. Or if your pain comes and goes, then do it whenever you happen to notice that the pain is there. Engaging with this exercise regularly, in a relaxed and genuinely curious way, will strengthen the brain's capacity to distinguish between a particular sensation and the emotions surrounding that sensation, which lays the groundwork for untangling the two experiences entirely.

Somatic Tracking

Of all the interventions that PRT practitioners use with their clients, the single most effective tool we use is somatic tracking (Gordon and Ziv 2021). Somatic tracking is, in many ways, the heart of PRT—it's the most powerful way we know to untangle sensation from fear, rewiring pain pathways so that neutral sensations no longer result in pain. It's a way of training your brain to gradually, over time, see a stump where it was once certain there stood a bear.

At its core, somatic tracking is about relating to your current physical experience with curious attention. If you already have some experience with mindfulness, aspects of somatic tracking will feel very familiar to you. But somatic tracking is not *just* mindfulness—it is mindfulness integrated with all of the work that you've already done to understand how pain works, to get to know your own nervous system, and to build and strengthen your foundation of safety. Indeed, both of your authors had extensive personal experience with mindfulness before coming into contact with PRT, and while mindfulness helped make our pain more tolerable at times, it wasn't until we began doing PRT that our chronic pain truly began to heal.

★ EXERCISE: Spaceman Somatic Tracking

One of the easiest ways to access the open and curious attitude of somatic tracking is by imagining that you are a spaceman exploring outer space. This metaphor might seem a little silly at first, but trust us, it's a great way to get into the explorer mindset that your brain needs to engage with sensations in a new way.

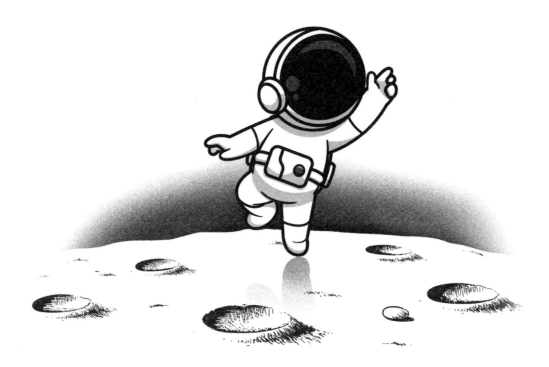

Figure 5.2 Spaceman

While you're experiencing pain, find a quiet space where you can have some privacy for at least twenty minutes. Take a relaxed posture, sitting or lying down, keeping in mind that physical discomfort is welcome in this exercise (there is no need to make yourself comfortable but also no need to make yourself any more uncomfortable than you need to be).

Close your eyes and imagine that you are a spaceman setting out to explore a new galaxy. This galaxy extends from the very top of your head to the very tips of your toes. Your job is to feel your way through the galaxy, sensation by sensation, getting to know it from the inside, so you can report back to the space station about what you find. Securely fasten your spaceman helmet, and settle in.

Use your internal awareness to scan this new galaxy from top to bottom, seeing what you discover along the way. As a result of past experience, you may have expectations about what you will find, but remember, even though this galaxy might remind you of ones you've visited before, this one is brand new—try to set your expectations aside in favor of being curious about what is actually there in this moment.

As you scan the body, where is the sensation most intense? What part of your body calls your attention most loudly? If more than one sensation is calling your attention, pick one—there is no such thing as a wrong answer. Bring your awareness to that sensation, and zoom in, feeling more deeply into the sensation to explore it further.

Letting your internal sense of touch do the thinking, what sensation words would you use to describe the sensation? Is it hard or soft? Tight or loose? Sharp or dull? Rough or smooth? Keep feeling into the sensation. How big is it right now? What shape is it in this moment? Do you feel any sense of pressure? If so, which direction is the pressure pushing—is it going in or out, front or back, left or right? Whatever you're experiencing, remember that it's just sensation—there is nothing to fear.

Continuing to explore, on a scale of 0 to 10, how unpleasant is this sensation? And now, on a scale of 0 to 10, how much distress about or resistance to sensation do you feel? Where in your body do you feel that distress or resistance?

Take a deep breath into the sensation. And breathe out. You're not trying to make the sensation go away or to change it in any way. You are simply breathing awareness into the sensation so you can feel it more clearly. With each inhale, feel your breath fill the sensation with awareness, then exhale naturally, allowing yourself to enjoy the feeling of air leaving your body. As you continue to breathe, allow your awareness to be relaxed and spacious—there is no need to catch every detail or to hold onto anything. Just be aware.

After five deep breaths like that, check back in with the sensation. What do you notice? Has it moved or changed in any way? Is it harder or softer than it was before? Sharper or duller? Rougher or smoother? On a scale of 0 to 10, how unpleasant is the sensation? And on a scale of 0 to 10, how much distress or resistance do you feel toward the sensation? Again, there is no right or wrong answer to any of these questions. Your only job is to notice what's happening, whatever that happens to be.

Can you find the epicenter of the sensation, that is, the place where it is most intense? If so, feel into that space. Now, use your awareness to find the very outer edge of the sensation, and feel into that. How does the outer edge compare to the epicenter? Is it harder or softer? Rougher or smoother? Tighter or looser? Warmer or cooler? Denser or more spacious? Whatever you discover, simply notice that's how it is right now.

Again, breathe deeply into the sensation, filling it with your awareness. You are not trying to control or change the sensation in any way—there is no need to fix. Just stay present with the *sensation, allowing it to do whatever it needs. You are a spaceman visiting this galaxy for the first time, and your only job is to observe what you find. Continue breathing into the sensation in this way.*

After five deep breaths, continue to explore the sensation. What do you notice now? Has the sensation moved or changed in some way? If so, how? If it hasn't moved or changed, notice that too. On a scale of 0 to 10, how unpleasant is the sensation? And on a scale of 0 to 10, how much distress or resistance do you feel toward the sensation?

Again, you're not looking for any particular answers here. You're just checking out the sensation as it is, whatever that may be. Is the sensation still or is it moving in some way? Is it pulsing, vibrating, or constant? If you notice pulsing, try to follow its rhythm for a minute or two by tapping on your chest every time you feel a pulse...tap, tap, tap.

Continue to explore the galaxy of your body in this way, attending to sensations that call your attention with genuine curiosity. If a sensation changes or moves, continue to track it as it transforms. Keep going like this. Remember, you aren't looking for anything special—no special result or magic moment. Rather, you're simply continuing to observe, allowing each sensation to do its thing, whatever that may be. With each moment that you attend to sensation in this way, you strengthen new neural pathways that make up the road to recovery.

When you are ready to stop, take off your spaceman helmet and store it somewhere safe for later, understanding that the next time you put it on, you will have a brand new galaxy to explore.

You did it. You had your first go at somatic tracking. As you practice, keep in mind that the particular characteristics of a given sensation—whether it is hard or soft, big or small, changing or constant, unpleasant or pleasant—are not important. Rather, you are inquiring about the sensations you're experiencing to shift your brain into curiosity mode, getting to know the sensation you are exploring in this moment as it actually is, whatever shape, size, or texture that may be. As you continue to engage with somatic tracking, you might experience painful sensations changing, becoming less intense, or maybe even fading away completely, but remember that decreasing the pain you're feeling right now is not the goal of somatic tracking. Rather, somatic tracking is about training your brain to relate to sensations through a lens of safety, interrupting the pain–fear cycle so that neuroplastic pain decreases in the long term. When you do somatic tracking, it's irrelevant whether the pain you're feeling right now goes away—what matters is that you're exploring it with genuine curiosity rather than trying to avoid or control it as you have in the past. This practice offers a new way of being in your body.

The more lighthearted and low stakes somatic tracking feels, the better, so feel free to be playful with it. In PRT, this is known as *positive affect induction* (Gordon and Ziv 2021). The more you can inject a sense of play or warmth—perhaps by imagining yourself as the adorable little spaceman—the easier it will be for your brain to relate to sensation through a lens of safety.

Don't worry about doing somatic tracking right or wrong—as long as you're exploring sensation with curiosity and through a lens of safety, you're doing your job. And as you get the hang of it, feel free to depart from the specifics set forth in the previously provided script, and let your curiosity be your guide. Continue to explore sensation in this curious and present-minded way in the months and years ahead. This new way of relating to sensation is a lifelong practice, and as with any new neural pathway, the more you practice, the easier it will get.

Special Instructions for Headache and Migraine

It's safe to say that your authors are passionate about headaches. We've both experienced migraines since childhood, and thanks to our own personal work with PRT, we know firsthand that debilitating headaches do not have to be a life sentence. Because head pain can be a little quirky, we want to offer a few special tips for using somatic tracking with headache and migraine:

Try somatic tracking even when you don't have a headache: While it's very worthwhile to do somatic tracking when you do have a headache, it's also worth engaging with somatic tracking when you don't. We've found that people who experience frequent headaches often have some sensation in or around the head or neck that is worth exploring, even if it hasn't yet risen to the level of a full-blown headache or migraine. Use somatic tracking to explore these more subtle sensations regularly, and see what you find. When exploring these sensations with curiosity, remember to assess not only how unpleasant the sensation is but also how much distress or resistance you feel toward them.

Breathe into your belly rather than the sensation itself: With most pain, the "Spaceman Somatic Tracking" exercise instructs you to explore breathing into the sensation itself. However, breathing into sensations in your head or neck can cause your breath to become quite shallow, which can inadvertently stimulate your sympathetic nervous system (danger mode). So, if you are working with sensations in your head or neck, try taking five deep belly breaths rather than breathing directly into the sensations themselves, then after five deep belly breaths, return your awareness to the sensations in your head or neck.

Be curious about sensory experiences you think of as "the beginning" of a migraine: Many of us have different sensory experiences that we have come to see as the first signs that a migraine is coming on—a tightness in the neck, throbbing at the temples, change in vision, or a particular taste on our tongues, to name a few. We habitually react to these signs with flavors of fear: dreading the migraine we know is coming, anxiously debating whether to take medication or not, worrying about the many ways this migraine will interfere with our plans for the day. But it's by responding to these signs with fear that we seal their fate. Often it's fear that transforms these so-called signs from harmless sensory experiences into full-blown migraines. So, next time you experience something you think of as "the beginning" of a migraine, use your somatic tracking skills to turn toward it and get curious. The more you can view these experiences through a lens of safety, the less likely they are to transform into the pain you've learned to fear.

Practice attending to sensation with somatic tracking regularly. If you only experience pain while standing or moving, you can do somatic tracking in those postures instead of the relaxed position described above. If you experience pain daily, we recommend trying spaceman-style somatic tracking once a day for at least ten days, as you are getting started. If you experience intermittent pain, try doing it only when you have pain, for a total of at least ten times. We know this is a big-time investment, but we promise you it's worth it. If you're going to be in pain, you might as well take the opportunity to strengthen these new neural pathways. Incorporating somatic tracking tips from the next section along the way, use the following practice log to record your observations about each of these early practice experiences. Record challenges you encounter, insights you experience, or questions that arise.

Somatic Tracking Practice Log	
1	
2	
3	
4	
5	
6	
7	
8	
9	
10	

Other Somatic Tracking Tips

As you practice somatic tracking, you might find that after so many years of relating to the familiar unpleasant sensations in your body with fear, it can take some time to get the hang of relating to old sensations in a new way. Here are some tips to help your brain make this transition:

Know When to Pivot

Somatic tracking's power to rewire your pain pathways depends on your brain's capacity to view sensations through a lens of safety. All brains have this natural capacity—yours too, we promise. But certain circumstances will make it easier for your brain to tap into that capacity than others. If your pain is through the roof, then it's going to be especially difficult for you to access a new perspective—and trying to push through when pain is high can actually reinforce your old pain pathways. So when pain is extreme, pivot. Shift your focus to other tools in your toolkit, like leaning into pleasant sensation or conjuring pleasant experience. Another time, when your pain is lower and the stakes don't feel quite so high, then you can turn your attention to somatic tracking. Similarly, you may find that twenty minutes of somatic tracking is far too long at first. For some nervous systems, a few minutes or even a few seconds may be the right amount to begin with. Give yourself permission to meet your nervous system where it is and trust that, in time, this gentle approach will prove far more beneficial for your healing than pushing through.

Tap into Your Foundation of Safety

Somatic tracking asks you to turn toward your pain, which can sometimes be a difficult leap for nervous systems that have spent so many years trying to avoid or control those same sensations. When doing somatic tracking, it's important to remind your brain that while the sensations you're experiencing may be mightily unpleasant, you are safe. In PRT this kind of reminder is known as a *safety reappraisal* (Gordon and Ziv 2021). Safety reappraisals are about tapping into your foundation of safety to help your overprotective nervous system relax enough to allow you to turn toward the sensations you're experiencing with genuine curiosity.

One way to incorporate safety reappraisals is by speaking directly to your own nervous system using your soothing self-talk tone. This is where your self-talk script or self-talk minis might come in. Safety reappraisals may also involve reflecting on the evidence that your own pain is neuroplastic to remind your brain that despite the unpleasant sensations you are experiencing, you are safe in this moment. You can also explore tapping into your foundation of safety in other ways by incorporating other tools from chapter 4 into the somatic tracking process. This might mean engaging with cold pack relaxation before you begin somatic tracking, or leaving the cold pack on your chest as you engage with it. While deep breathing is already incorporated into the "Spaceman Somatic Tracking" exercise, you may find that you want to extend these periods, leaning into the pleasant experience of breathing for ten or twenty breaths instead of just five.

If your protective parts are activated in the course of somatic tracking, remember that you don't need to make those parts disappear or go away. You just want to help them feel safe enough to give you some space to explore sensation in a new way. If you find that, even after tapping into your foundation of safety, your protective parts are still unwilling to take a step back, honor that—take a break from somatic tracking and dedicate some time to soothing your nervous system in other ways. Go for a walk outside, get together with a friend, or watch a good movie. If and when down the line you find that your protective parts feel relaxed enough to give you some space, then you can return to somatic tracking and give it another go.

Acknowledge and Attend to Feelings of Distress

Sometimes, as you engage in somatic tracking, you might notice that feelings of distress or resistance are notably more intense than the unpleasantness of the sensation itself. Perhaps you notice that the unpleasantness of a particular sensation is a 6 out of 10, but your distress about that sensation (or your resistance to it) is a 9 out of 10. In this case, where distress or resistance is so prominent, take some time to explore the distress itself by shifting your awareness from the original sensation you were exploring to your feelings of distress about that sensation. Notice where you feel the distress in your body and bring your awareness there, feeling into it and exploring that feeling in the same way that you would use somatic tracking to explore any other sensation. Attend to the feeling of distress with the same curiosity you would devote to any other sensation in your body. If and when that distress fades or diminishes so it's no longer so prominent, bring your awareness back to the original sensation to continue somatic tracking.

Be Mindful of Intensity, Perfectionism, Control, and Self-Judgment

If you notice intensity, perfectionism, control, or self-judgment creeping in as you engage with somatic tracking, these are some of the more subtle ways that your nervous system might be trying to protect you. Alas, when you engage with somatic tracking when intensity, perfectionism, control, or self-judgment are at the wheel, your brain won't have an opportunity to perceive sensations as they really are.

Luckily, you don't need to change your whole personality to do somatic tracking. You can be an intense perfectionist who is prone to control and self-judgment and still recover from neuroplastic pain—we promise! The key is to simply be mindful of these old habits when they arise. Use NABS from chapter 3—notice, acknowledge, befriend, and shift—to work with your protective parts rather than against them. So, for example, as you engage with somatic tracking, *notice* when you are doing so in a particularly intense way: perhaps you are tracking sensations with a laser focus, watching them like a hawk. If that happens, simply *acknowledge* it: *Oh, there's intensity again, trying to make sure I give my all.* There's no need to fight this old habit of intensity. Instead, *befriend* it: remind yourself that this old habit is just trying to protect you, and let the old habit know that although you're trying a new way of doing things, it's more than welcome to come along for the ride. Finally, *shift* into a new, more relaxed mode, zooming out from the sensations you're exploring, so you can observe them in a looser, more spacious way, as you might gaze at the flames in a campfire or at clouds passing by overhead.

Similarly, if you notice a sense of hypervigilance about doing somatic tracking perfectly, acknowledge, *Oh wow, there's perfectionism, trying to make sure that I do this just right.* Thank perfectionism for everything it has done to try to protect you: it has worked so hard for so long to keep you safe, and this is just one more example of it trying to do just that. Then, without getting into a wrestling match with perfectionism, simply shift into a new low-stakes way of doing things: remind yourself that you're totally safe right now and that it can take a little while to get the hang of somatic tracking. It can take some time to learn this new way of relating to sensations, and it might not come easily at first, but so long as you keep practicing, you'll get the hang of it eventually, because that's what brains do.

If you notice that a part of you is trying to control the sensation or fix it in some way, gently acknowledge, *There's my old friend control, working so hard to make sure that everything turns out okay.* Befriend it, understanding where this old habit comes from and how much it cares. Then, shift: even if only for a few moments, give yourself permission to loosen your grip.

Finally, if you notice self-judgment coming up—maybe in the form of critical self-talk or being hard on your protective parts for getting in the way—there's no need to judge the self-judgment. Just acknowledge, *Oh, look, there's self-judgment working really hard to keep me on track*, and then practice treating that self-judgment with kindness and even thanking it for everything it's been trying to do to help you get better. There's no need to fight the old habit of self-judgment when it arises—just see it as another opportunity to shift into your new habit of self-kindness.

Use NABS whenever you notice a protective part trying to grab the wheel. And, if a part is not willing to step back, respect that. Take this as an opportunity to strengthen your relationship with that part by using the "Getting to Know Your Inner Protectors" exercise from chapter 3.

Notice When Outcome Dependence Is in the Driver's Seat

One of the sneakiest ways that your protective parts can take the wheel is by engaging with somatic tracking in an effort to make the pain you're feeling right now go away. As we emphasized at the beginning of this book, outcome independence is important on the road to recovery. You need to put one foot in front of the other without attachment to a particular outcome. The opposite of that approach is *outcome dependence*—that is, engaging with your tools to bring about a particular result. Of course you want your pain to decrease—that's the whole reason you're doing this workbook, right? But, when you do somatic tracking in an effort to make the pain you're feeling *right now* go away, this agenda undercuts the whole process: the urgent desire to decrease your pain reinforces the brain's belief that the pain is threatening in some way. This not only gets in the way of your brain perceiving sensation through a lens of safety but actually pours more fuel on the fire of the pain–fear cycle.

There's nothing wrong with wanting your pain to go away—it's the most natural desire there is. So when you discover that outcome dependence is in the driver's seat—and you will!—what the heck do you do about it? Again, turn to NABS for support. Once you've noticed that you're doing somatic tracking with the agenda of making the pain you're observing decrease, take a moment to acknowledge it: *Oh, hey, look—there's my brain trying to make the pain go away.* Rather than struggling with this protective habit, befriend it. Take a few moments to reflect on how natural it is to want to feel better and how anyone in your position would want the same thing. Let this part of your brain know that you want to feel better too, and thank it for everything it's trying to do to help. Then, ask it if it would be willing to sit in the backseat for just a few minutes as you try out this new way of relating to sensation. Once your brain's focus on outcome has relaxed a bit, return to the somatic tracking script. If, along the way, you notice outcome dependence sneaking back into the driver's seat, just gently notice, acknowledge, befriend, and shift. It might take some time, but eventually your brain will begin to trust that this new, more relaxed way of relating to sensation is not only safe but onward leading.

Be Aware of the Stories Your Brain Tells

Many of us have stories that we've told about our pain for a long time. Sometimes, these stories stem from our own (very understandable) efforts to make sense of the pain we've been feeling—stories about getting headaches when the atmospheric pressure changes or nausea when we're around perfumes or back pain when it's cold. And sometimes these stories have been told to us by health care providers along the way: the pinched nerve in your shoulder, the bulging disc in your spine, or the "bone on bone" arthritis in your ankle. Often, these stories are accompanied by images we've seen—CT scans, MRIs, and X-rays—and other times these stories are accompanied by images that our brains have created based on what we understand to be happening in our bodies. But no matter where these stories and images originally come from, they are likely to get in the way of your brain's capacity to perceive sensation as it really is, because they are telling your brain what it should expect to feel.

Due to predictive coding, which we discussed earlier in this chapter, the stories that your brain uses to explain the sensations you're experiencing—and the images that accompany those stories—will, in turn, play a role in creating those sensations. So, if a doctor explained your back pain by pointing to the bulging disc in your MRI, then you are likely to *feel* a bulging disc in your back, whatever your brain interprets that to mean. The more attached you are to specific stories and images surrounding sensation, the stickier those sensations will be.

You don't need to completely disbelieve these stories to heal. After all, you may very well have a bulging disc in your back! But, as many people who have had success with PRT will tell you, having a bulging disc does not necessarily mean that you need to be in pain. While there may or may not be something going on in your body, the pain is coming from your brain. Give your brain permission to loosen its grip on the story it tells about the pain you experience, and get curious about what it actually feels.

The key here is to let your sense of touch do the thinking, as you learned to do in the first exercise in this chapter. If you are doing somatic tracking, and you find yourself describing the sensation you're exploring as "feeling like a pinched nerve" or "feeling like two bones are rubbing against each other," notice that those are stories your brain is telling about the sensations you're experiencing rather than the sensations themselves. Allow your brain to set the story aside for now, and feel the sensation as it actually is rather than through the lens of your old beliefs about *why* it is.

Advanced Somatic Tracking

Once you've done the "Spaceman Somatic Tracking" exercise at least ten times, giving your brain the chance to strengthen those open and curious neural pathways, you can drop the spaceman narrative if you like and move on to the simplified version of somatic tracking presented here.

★ EXERCISE: Simple Somatic Tracking

Try this simpler version of somatic tracking. If at any point you find that your brain needs a bit more support, remember that your spaceman helmet is always there to help you reconnect with your inner explorer when you need it.

Close your eyes and bring your awareness to whatever part of your body is calling your attention most loudly. Feel into that space as if for the very first time, and let your sense of touch do the thinking. How big is the sensation? What shape is it? What sensation words would you use to describe it?

Do you feel any sense of pressure? If so, which direction is the pressure going—in or out, front or back, left or right?

On a scale of 0 to 10, how unpleasant is the sensation? And, on a scale of 0 to 10, how much distress about or resistance to the sensation do you feel?

Feel into the very epicenter of the sensation. Now, feel into the very outside edge of the sensation. How would you compare the two?

Continue to explore. Is the sensation moving or changing in any way? Is it vibrating, pulsing, or totally still? Continue to stay present with the sensation, observing, as it does whatever it needs to do.

Gently hold the sensation in the palm of your awareness. There is no need to fix or control the sensation. Just observe. Whatever you're experiencing, it's just sensation—there is nothing to fear.

You'll notice that this version does not specifically instruct you to breathe into the sensation. While we've found that including breathing in a structured way can be quite helpful when you're first getting the hang of somatic tracking, as you get more familiar with the practice, we leave it up to you if and when you want to incorporate breath.

As you continue to practice somatic tracking, you may also find that the various questions—"How big is the sensation?" "What sensation words would you use to describe it?" "On a scale of 1 to 10, how unpleasant is the sensation?"—begin to feel unnecessary. Think of these questions like training wheels: there early on to help your brain get the hang of relating to sensation in this radically new way. As you continue to practice, your brain will need them less and less. If you find that you're able to stay present with sensation without using questions, then do that. If it feels like your brain is starting to hold on a little too tightly—trying to control the sensation or push it away—drop in a few of your favorite somatic tracking questions to help it get back on track. Remember, there is no right or wrong here. Just keep exploring, and neuroplasticity will take care of the rest.

The somatic tracking scripts in this chapter are here to support you as you develop your somatic tracking skills. But somatic tracking doesn't need to be a big formal event. As you continue to practice, you'll eventually reach a place where relating to sensations in this way starts to feel totally natural, even automatic. When you find yourself there, allow yourself to drop the scripts altogether, and simply let curiosity be your guide. If and when you find that your brain needs a booster, return to the scripts. And remember, there is no sensation too big for awareness.

Next Steps

In this chapter, you've begun to transform your relationship with sensation. You've learned to let your sense of touch do the thinking and to turn this capacity inward to untangle sensation from the fear around the sensation. In the next chapter, you'll learn to extend this same curious and open approach to the whole of your inner life, including the experience of fear itself.

CHAPTER 6

The Path Forward

Welcome to the final chapter. Stay here for a moment, taking in the remarkable journey your brain has traversed since the start of this workbook. In the opening chapters, you peeled back the layers of neuroplastic pain, digging into its mysteries and discovering fear's starring role. Then, as you journeyed forward, you and your nervous system became allies. A new awareness blossomed, revealing how the pain–fear cycle shows up in your own mind and body. Step by step, you laid the foundation for a more resilient nervous system. And with your bedrock of safety fortified, you turned toward the pain itself, learning to view painful sensations through a lens of safety rather than a lens of danger.

This final chapter is the culmination of your journey. Here, your brain continues on its mission to perceive sensations through a lens of safety, learning to extend the attentive and curious approach you've learned to take toward physical sensation to all aspects of your internal experience, including the sensations associated with emotions themselves. Safety doesn't always mean everything is pristine and perfect. What it does mean is that, even amid stress and worry, your body is no longer sabotaging you. You're providing your brain with a new set of glasses, ones that see neutral sensations for what they truly are: harmless. You're also learning to see yourself as more capable than your experience with neuroplastic pain has led you to believe. Repeat after us: "I am not as fragile as I fear I am."

This chapter will guide you in learning to turn toward your internal state rather than away from it. The more adept your brain becomes at viewing your inner world through this lens of safety, the more finely tuned its discernment between harmless and dangerous sensations will grow. As a consequence, the grip of neuroplastic pain loosens, paving the way for a future with diminished pain and increased well-being.

Exploring Emotion Through a Lens of Safety

Because our brains can—as a result of life experiences—become conditioned to respond to certain emotions with fear, emotions have the power to trigger neuroplastic pain. For this reason, learning to relate to your emotions through a lens of safety is an important component of pain recovery.

EXERCISE: Feeling Your Feelings

There's a good reason that the other word for emotions is "feelings"—we *feel* emotions in our bodies. Sadness may show up as a tightness in the throat, anxiety as pressure in the chest, or anger as a burning in the belly. All emotional experience is accompanied by physical sensation, although just how and where it shows up will vary from person to person.

Emotion-related sensations can be quite subtle, and many of us are not aware of them at all, but whether you're aware of them or not, they're there. For many people who experience neuroplastic symptoms, the relationship between emotion and pain got scrambled somewhere along the way, and the brain began to misinterpret emotion-related sensations as signs of danger. If you're one of those people, particular emotions might trigger pain without you even knowing it. By learning to feel your feelings, your brain will begin to recognize emotions for what they are: harmless sensory experiences that absolutely need your care and attention but are not threats to your physical safety.

This emotion wheel includes a broad range of emotions that you might feel in your daily life. To help your brain become more acquainted with how emotions feel in your body, use the log provided to record three emotions per day over the next week. For each emotion, write down where you feel it in your body and at least one sensation word to describe how it feels. Although you are welcome to repeat emotions from day to day, we encourage you to keep an eye out for new emotions to expand your body's emotional vocabulary as much as possible.

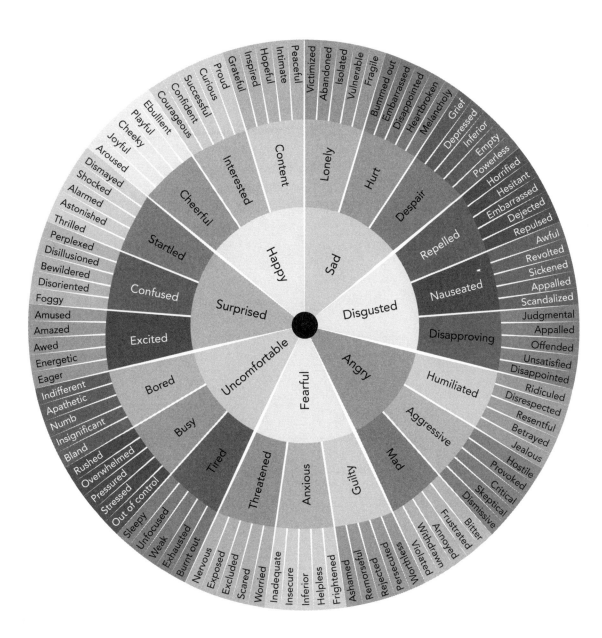

Figure 6.1 Emotion Wheel

Day	Emotion	Where in Body?	Sensation?
1			
2			
3			
4			
5			
6			
7			

This exercise allowed you to begin touching into the way emotions show up in your body. The next exercise takes this a step further, focusing on one emotion at a time and going deeper. Here you will practice applying your somatic tracking skills directly to the felt experience of emotion itself.

★ EXERCISE: Somatic Tracking Emotion

Find a comfortable, quiet space where you won't be disturbed for at least twenty minutes. Take a relaxed posture, either sitting or lying down.

Step 1: Refer to Spaceman Somatic Tracking

When you're entering into this emotion exploration, we encourage you to use the same curious mindset that was established in chapter 5 in the "Spaceman Somatic Tracking" exercise. Secure your spaceman helmet, take a deep breath, and settle in.

Step 2: Identify the Dominant Emotion

Scan your emotional galaxy. What emotion is calling your attention most loudly? Use the emotion wheel to guide you, or feel free to identify an emotion not included there. There's no wrong answer. Write down the emotion you've chosen to explore:

Step 3: Zoom In

Focus on that emotion. Locate where you feel it in your body. What does it feel like? Is it heavy or light, warm or cool, contracted or expansive? Use the sensation words you learned in the last chapter, and allow your sense of touch to do the thinking. With these sensations as your focal point, engage with the full "Spaceman Somatic Tracking" exercise from chapter 5, tracking these emotion-related sensations in the same way that you would track any others.

Step 4: Closure

When you're ready to conclude, acknowledge the journey. Take off your spaceman helmet, knowing that each time you put it on, the emotional galaxy you encounter will be entirely brand new.

Step 5: Reflect and Integrate

Write a brief reflection on your experience during this activity. Note any shifts in your perspective, feelings, or attitudes toward your emotions.

_____

_____

_____

_____

As you continue this practice, let curiosity be your guide. Explore emotions with openness and kindness, fostering a deeper understanding of your emotional terrain. Remember, the goal is not to change or control emotions but to observe and build a resilient relationship with them. As you grow more familiar with relating to emotion in this way, you can follow the same trajectory that you did in chapter 5, moving on to a simpler version of somatic tracking and eventually going completely off script and letting your own curiosity be your guide.

This is a lifelong practice, and the more you engage, the more familiar and comfortable you'll become with your emotional galaxy. The more your brain learns to view emotions through a lens of safety, the less likely it will be to misinterpret them as dangerous and the less pain you will feel.

Imaginal Exposure

The brain is a masterful creator, capable of translating thoughts, fears, and expectations into palpable sensations. Neuroplastic pain represents one, less helpful way that this tendency can manifest. There are also more helpful ones, like the practice of "provocative testing," a technique created by Dr. Howard Schubiner, MD, which involves using your imagination to explore situations that might cause pain (Schubiner and Betzold 2022). By doing this, you bring these situations to mind and observe whether your brain reacts with pain. If pain arises in the absence of the actual physical situation, this validates a link between your thoughts and the pain experience, helping you understand the psychological aspects of your pain.

Similarly, in the practice of imaginal exposure, a person vividly imagines a distressing stimulus, so they can contact their anxiety and begin to work with it, learning that while anxiety can be intense, it's not dangerous. Here, we offer your brain the opportunity to harness the power of imagination to heal. As you embark on this activity, the goal is to unravel the connection between your thought patterns and the body's response. By immersing yourself in this practice, you pave the way for greater awareness and, ultimately, transformation.

EXERCISE: Unraveling Distress

Is there a task or situation you've been steering clear of because of the distress it stirs within you or the physical pain it triggers? Take a moment to jot it down.

_____

_____

Vividly imagine this distressing scenario, allowing your mind to paint a detailed picture. Feel the emotions that surface as you navigate this mental landscape. What flavors of fear do you notice? Are there other emotions present as well?

_____

_____

Now, employing the art of somatic tracking, turn your attention inward toward the sensations you're experiencing. Explore these sensations using the same approach outlined in the previous exercise. Without judgment, let your sense of touch do the thinking. Delve into the nuances of these bodily responses, observing how they ebb and flow with the contours of your emotions. What do you notice?

_____

_____

As you engage with this exercise, you may notice that your distress intensifies. That's okay. Just stick with it, and continue to stay present with the understanding that some emotions get more intense before they fade away. Your job is to simply attend to whatever arises.

Exploring Urgency

Now that you have explored your emotions with more curiosity, we'd like to focus on one particular emotional experience that often crops up for people with neuroplastic pain: a sense of urgency that guides your reactions. For example, do you ever feel the need to react right away, even when it might not be necessary? It's a common experience, but not always helpful. Urgency tends to pop up from ingrained habits rather than real demands. It's like your brain has an automatic "react now" setting. But here's the twist: not every situation requires urgent action. In fact, jumping into action without thinking can sometimes make things worse.

Urgency often manifests as a heightened state of readiness or pressure to act quickly. Here are some signs and sensations that may indicate a sense of urgency in your mind and body:

Mental restlessness: You might experience a racing mind, where thoughts are rapid or jump from one idea to another. There's a sense of mental urgency to figure things out or make decisions swiftly.

Physical tension: Urgency can manifest as physical tension in the body. You may feel tightness in your muscles, especially in the shoulders, neck, or jaw. This tension can be a response to the perceived need for immediate action.

Increased heart rate: A faster heartbeat is a common physiological response to urgency, as if your body is gearing up for a rapid response.

Shallow breathing: When urgency kicks in, breathing may become shallower and more rapid. This can contribute to a feeling of restlessness and further amplify the overall sense of urgency.

Sense of pressure: You might feel a sense of pressure or a deadline looming even if there isn't one. This pressure can prompt you to take action to relieve the perceived stress.

Impatience: Feeling impatient or a strong desire for things to happen quickly is another aspect of urgency. It's a sense of wanting immediate results or resolution.

Difficulty relaxing: Urgency can make it challenging to relax or engage in activities that require patience. There's a nagging feeling that time is of the essence.

By being aware of these indicators, you can start to recognize when urgency is present in your mind and body. This awareness is the first step in developing a more mindful and measured approach to situations that trigger urgency, allowing you to respond with greater clarity and intention.

How Urgency Becomes the Norm

You may be able to easily recall a scenario where urgency was a constant companion. Perhaps you've faced challenging circumstances that demanded quick decisions and immediate action, fostering a belief that urgency is the norm. Take Vanessa's experience, for example. Her brain simply adapted to chaos and urgency out of survival, leading to an overprotective nervous system that seemed to be missing its off button. If your past experiences were marked by a genuine need for urgency, your brain may have adapted to this pattern in the same way Vanessa's did, perceiving urgency as a valid and necessary response. This adaptation served you well in navigating circumstances where rapid decisions were crucial for survival.

Does this describe your experience? Take some time to name experiences you've had where your sense of urgency protected you from harm.

_____

_____

The challenge arises when this learned sense of urgency persists even in situations that don't pose an immediate threat. If you've lived through urgent circumstances before, it's understandable that your brain might default to this mode, applying it broadly to your everyday experiences. The key lies in recognizing that not every situation requires an urgent response, allowing your brain the space to discern between genuine emergencies and situations where a more measured approach is appropriate. By gaining insight into the origins of this automatic response, you can start to untangle the threads of urgency from your past, and reframe your approach to current challenges. By learning to relate to urgency in this new way, you pave the way for a more intentional and balanced response to the world around you.

The next exercise is designed to help you observe the sense of urgency when it arises. As you engage with it, pay close attention to the physical sensations associated with urgency. Notice if there's a tendency to urgently notice the urgency itself! The essence of this exercise is to allow the sense of urgency to unfold without succumbing to its demands. Resist the impulse to act immediately in response to the sense of urgency. Instead, give yourself permission to witness urgency's presence, allowing it to arise, strengthen, and gradually dissipate all on its own.

EXERCISE: Riding the Waves of Urgency

Think back on a recent experience, sometime in the last week, when you experienced a sign of urgency that wasn't so useful and maybe even harmed more than it helped. What was happening, where were you, and what did it feel like?

_____

_____

_____

_____

When that spike in urgency finally dissipated, what was left? What did your body feel like?

_____

_____

_____

_____

What tool, reminder, or skill would you like to use to respond differently the next time you notice a sign of urgency?

_____

_____

_____

_____

By refraining from doing what the sense of urgency compels you to do, you prevent the reinforcement of habitual patterns. This exercise invites a practice of nonreactivity, allowing you to break the cycle of urgency-driven responses.

Over time, as you integrate this awareness into your daily life, you'll strengthen a newfound capacity to navigate stressful situations with greater ease and resilience.

Attending to Your Internal State

Pausing to attend to your internal state allows you to step out of autopilot mode, creating a space for awareness and self-reflection, which enables you to break free from the habitual responses that fuel pain. This is why taking a moment to pause and check in with what's happening in your own body and mind is a foundational practice of PRT. In the hustle of daily life, we often overlook subtle cues that our minds and bodies provide. The next exercise is designed to help you recognize the thoughts, feelings, and behaviors that signal the need for a pause.

EXERCISE: Identifying Your Meditation Bells

We all have our own unique signs that indicate when our overprotective nervous systems are kicking into gear. Imagine each of these signs is a meditation bell, gently reminding you to take some time to attend to your internal state.

One person's meditation bell might be slipping into detective mode, obsessively seeking answers to *why* you're feeling the way you feel. For another, it might be getting stuck in fix-it mind, urgently seeking solutions to make whatever challenge you're experiencing go away, once and for all. And for another, it may be as simple as a physical sensation—perhaps a familiar pressure in the chest, tightness in the throat, or a pinch between the eyebrows. Alternatively, it could be a particular tone in your voice or a specific way that your shoulders hunch over when you're stressed. Whatever these signs are for you, take a few minutes to identify them here.

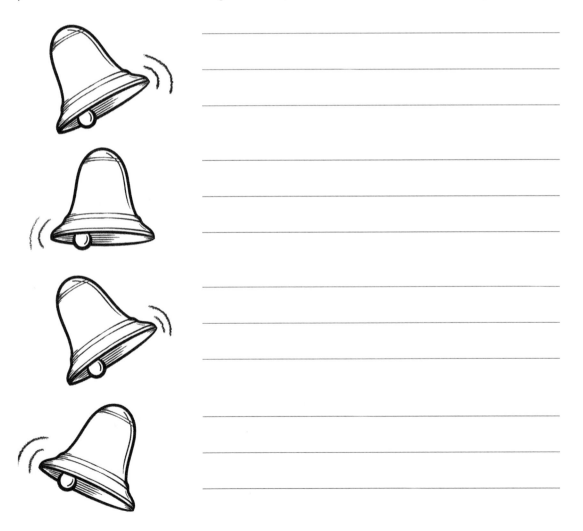

By recognizing your meditation bells, you gain the power to interrupt these automatic responses, fostering a more balanced and mindful approach to your internal experiences.

Exploring Body Positions and Movements Through a Lens of Safety

Certain behaviors can prompt your brain to declare, *Alert, danger ahead!* Behaviors can be the positions we assume while lying, sitting, or standing; movements and transitions, which can be associated with what is known as *transitional pain*; and specific activities associated with pain.

We want to introduce you to a chronic pain sufferer whom we will call "Jake," another client at the Pain Psychology Center. Jake initially grappled with discomfort localized in his right knee, especially after running. He assumed it was a straightforward running injury, perhaps a ligament tear. Taking the logical step, he ceased running. However, a surprising twist awaited him: standing gradually evolved into a challenge. Believing orthotics might hold the key, Jake embraced that solution. Unfortunately, the relief was short-lived, and eventually, being upright in any way triggered pain. As time elapsed, sitting also transformed into a source of agony. Fast forward six years, and Jake found himself entangled in a complex web involving twenty different medical professionals, two surgeries, six medications, dozens of physical therapy sessions, and a myriad of other specialists. The knee pain that began with running had morphed into sharp sensations in his left hip, radiating up his back and persistently throbbing throughout the day. Despite extensive medical interventions, Jake's symptoms persisted, leading him to reach out to the Pain Psychology Center as a final resort.

In chapter 2, we described how flavors of fear amplify pain signals—paradoxically, your attempts to shield yourself from pain, while rooted in a survival instinct, can inadvertently exacerbate the very pain you seek to avoid. Healing is, in part, a matter of persuading the brain to shed its armor, assuring it that safety is attainable without such defensive measures. In the realm of behaviors, one flavor of fear is especially important: avoidance. It is natural to avoid the behavior you believe is causing your pain, but what if the pain isn't actually caused by the behavior itself? What if, instead, it results from your brain's belief that the behavior is perilous when, in reality, it isn't?

To help answer that question, we will introduce you to another chronic pain sufferer whom we'll call "Kat," also a client at the Pain Psychology Center. Diagnosed with rheumatoid arthritis (RA) in 2002, Kat's journey was marked by a relentless escalation of pain since their initial diagnosis. From the outset, the diagnosis cast a shadow over their future. Kat came to expect pain and the limitations that came with it: a long list of activities that their body "couldn't" handle, countless rules and recommendations to follow, and an endless cycle of symptom management. For Kat, a core challenge lay in identifying specific behaviors that triggered symptoms. Triggering behaviors were everywhere: putting on a shirt, bending to retrieve a fallen object, opening a sliding glass door to let out their dogs, and descending stairs (although, curiously, ascending stairs posed no issue). The interesting twist was that—despite triggers at every turn—Kat was still fairly mobile. Working long hours, taking care of their home, and maintaining a family life wasn't always comfortable, but they could manage it. While Kat's RA diagnosis was substantiated by imaging, they experienced a lingering determination to explore avenues beyond conventional symptom management. This commitment to live life beyond the bounds of their diagnosis is what prompted Kat to reach out to the Pain Psychology Center for support.

Before going further into Jake and Kat's transformative journeys, explore your own relationship with triggering behaviors in the exercise below.

★ EXERCISE: Navigating Behaviors and Sensations

Here, we invite you to turn toward those behaviors that have historically triggered pain. To recall a previous example, for Olivia this was any aerobic exercise that increased her heart rate. For you, it could be sitting for extended periods, standing for too long, walking, or any other activity that has become associated with discomfort.

Once you've identified a triggering behavior, you'll apply your somatic tracking skills to view that behavior—and the sensations associated with it—through a lens of safety. The goal here is not to endure unnecessary pain but to approach triggering behaviors with mindful awareness.

Step 1: Choose a Triggering Behavior

Select a specific behavior that tends to provoke pain or discomfort. This could be a behavioral trigger that you identified in the "Pain Maps" exercise in chapter 3 or something else entirely:

Step 2: Prepare for the Activity

Before engaging in your chosen behavior, take a moment to connect with your foundation of safety. Breathe deeply, acknowledging any apprehension, anxiety, or other flavors of fear. If you notice any protective parts stepping into the driver's seat, practice NABS, and ask your protective parts if they'd be willing to give you some space for a few minutes while you engage with this exercise. Remind yourself that this is an exploration, not a test or an endurance challenge.

Step 3: Engage Mindfully

Once you've connected with your foundation of safety, begin to engage with your chosen behavior. As you do so, notice any changes in your body, both subtle and pronounced, as well as changes in your emotions and thoughts. Practice observing your experience without judgment.

Step 4: Use Somatic Tracking

As sensations arise—whether they are unpleasant, pleasant, or neutral—employ the somatic tracking skills you've learned in this workbook to stay present with your physical experience. Check in with the parts of your body that call your attention most loudly, turning toward any tension or discomfort with curiosity. Continue on like this for some time, attending to your internal state through a lens of safety.

Step 5: Record Your Observations

Keep a journal or make mental notes of what you observe during the activity. Document insights, shifts in perception, or challenges you encounter along the way.

Step 6: Reflect on Emotions

After completing the activity, take a moment to reflect on the emotions that surfaced during the process. What flavors of fear did you notice? How did these emotions correlate with the physical sensations you experienced?

_____

_____

_____

_____

Step 7: Practice Self-Compassion

Regardless of the outcome, be kind to yourself. This exercise is not about pushing boundaries but about cultivating awareness. Recognize any progress, no matter how small, and acknowledge the courage it took to engage in this exploration.

_____

_____

Remember, the goal of this exercise is not to make the pain go away. Rather, it's to practice viewing whatever sensations you experience—whether painful or otherwise—through a lens of safety. Each time you do this, you weaken the association between the chosen behavior and pain, taking another step on the road of recovery.

Returning to our earlier stories about Jake and Kat, both triumphed over their chronic pain, and changing the way that they related to their historically identified triggers was key for both of them. For Jake, the road to recovery was a gradual process. It took time for him to recognize that his knee pain was a symptom of his distress rather than the cause of it. He came to understand that neuroplastic pain wasn't his brain's attempt to sabotage him. Rather, it was signaling a need for change in his life: a true reckoning with emotionally taxing relationships and the burdens of parenthood, among other chronic stressors. Ultimately, Jake used the techniques you've learned to reshape the way his brain relates to sensation. He learned to turn toward triggering emotions and behaviors rather than away from them, enabling his brain to shift from viewing these experiences through a lens of danger to viewing them through a lens of safety. As he grew more attuned to his internal experience, his journey toward healing also came to involve shedding those aspects of his life that persistently eroded his sense of safety. By using these tools with patience, persistence, and compassion, Jake lit the path to his own recovery.

Kat's epiphany came when they realized their body did not need to be defined by a scary diagnosis. Yes, they had RA, but it didn't need to rule their body or life. Fueled by this insight, Kat turned toward their trigger behaviors with curiosity. By looking closely at their internal experience, Kat was able to witness firsthand the way in which fear amplified their pain, and suddenly each painful sensation was seen for the false alarm it was. Seeing through this illusion, Kat was genuinely delighted, and the more Kat laughed, the more empowered they felt. By learning to exhale into the transition of movement rather than perpetually bracing for pain, Kat gave themself permission to stop fighting their nervous system and start working with it. This breakthrough paved the way for liberating them to feel free in their body.

The following exercise encourages you to identify tools you can use to decrease fear and effectively break the chains holding you back from a more liberated and pain-free life. The goal is to disrupt old patterns by intentionally introducing new, positive behaviors that serve to decrease fear.

EXERCISE: Breaking the Chain

Use this strategy to rewire neural pathways associated with pain.

Step 1: Review Your Pain Maps

Take a moment to revisit the pain maps you created in chapter 3. Identify specific points in the maps you created where behaviors—activities, postures, movements, and so on—trigger pain responses.

Choose one behavior that consistently leads to discomfort:

Step 2: Brainstorm

Brainstorm a few different ways that you can decrease the fear response that's triggered by the behavior you've identified. For example, when Olivia was out on a run and noticed familiar old flavors of fear arising—like the habit of repeatedly checking on the sensations in her head to see if pain had started—she would interrupt that response by intentionally bringing her attention elsewhere, using the brain game of listening to all the sounds she could discover around her (see the section in chapter 4 on playing with preoccupation). You can list any of the fear-reducing tools you've learned in this book or any other tricks you've picked up that help to interrupt the fear response.

_____

_____

_____

Step 3: Choose New Behaviors

Select one or two fear-reducing tools that especially resonate with you. These should be actions you can integrate into your daily life to interrupt fear when it arises in response to triggering behaviors.

Begin incorporating the new tools into your daily life when flavors of fear arise, starting gradually in order to allow your brain to adapt. Be patient with yourself as you navigate this transition. The goal is to build new associations and responses over time.

_____

_____

Step 4: Document Your Progress

Note any shifts in your pain experience, however small. Celebrate successes and use challenges as opportunities for learning and adjustment.

_____

_____

Remember, breaking the chain is a dynamic process, and the goal is not perfection but progress. This exercise empowers you to actively participate in reshaping your neural pathways and promoting a more positive relationship between behaviors and pain.

Healing Is Not Linear

Healing is a nuanced journey filled with twists and turns, and understanding that it's not a linear process is essential for your progress. In the world of pain recovery, there are usually times when the pain pops up again after a period of apparent progress. Whether you call it a setback, relapse, flare-up, or hitting a wall, it's crucial to distinguish what's actually happening from what you fear is happening. Whatever you've called it before, the phrase used here is *extinction burst*.

An extinction burst occurs when symptoms intensify temporarily after a period of decline. It's the flare-up you experience just when it seemed like things were finally starting to get better (Gordon and Ziv 2021). Extinction bursts occur because old neural pathways have a momentum all their own and don't give up without a fight. For quite a while now, pain has been your nervous system's go-to strategy in its tenacious effort to protect you, and extinction bursts happen when your brain is afraid that it's losing its capacity to keep you safe. Note that symptoms can be quite intense during these periods and are often even more severe than they were before you began to recover. Your task is simply to see extinction bursts clearly for what they are and to respond with patience and compassion rather than fear.

Before you came to understand that extinction bursts are a natural part of the healing process, you most likely misinterpreted the flare-ups you've experienced in the course of this workbook as evidence of backsliding. Take a moment to think about the last time you experienced a flare-up. What happened, where were you, and what went through your mind? What flavors of fear did you experience? Rest your eyebrows, part your teeth, and reflect with a few natural breaths. When you're ready, describe that event:

_____

_____

_____

_____

_____

_____

_____

_____

_____

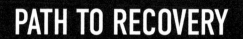

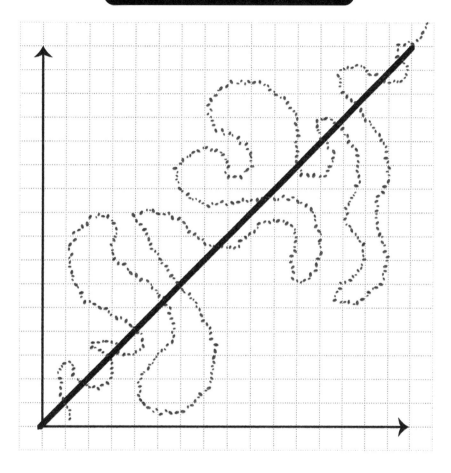

WHAT PEOPLE THINK HEALING LOOKS LIKE ━━━━━━━━━

WHAT HEALING ACTUALLY LOOKS LIKE ●●●●●●●●●●●●●●

Figure 6.3 Path to Recovery

Now that you understand what extinction bursts are, your task is to accept them as a natural part of the healing process. Sure, they can be unpleasant, but so long as you view them through a lens of safety, they don't need to be any more than that. Harnessing the power of outcome independence, use your tools in the same way you have before, with curiosity, patience, and compassion. Each extinction burst you experience is just another opportunity to strengthen your new neural pathways. With that in mind, keep putting one foot in front of the other and trust the process.

While we think that was a pretty good pep talk, we know from experience that the most powerful pep talk is the one you give yourself. Wait to engage with this next exercise until a moment when you're feeling particularly confident about your own capacity for recovery. When that moment arises, return to this workbook and focus on the confidence you're feeling. Maybe you're feeling confident because your pain faded away when you did somatic tracking…or because your symptoms have been noticeably less intense for the last few days…or because you engaged in a behavior you used to avoid, only to discover it didn't cause so much discomfort after all. Whatever the reason, use this positive mindset to guide you in this letter-writing exercise. When challenging times come along, you can return to this letter to keep your perspective and stay the course.

EXERCISE: Reflective Letter Writing

Begin by finding a quiet and comfortable space with your journal or writing paper. Date the letter and address it to yourself. Start by reviewing and answering the following prompts.

Acknowledge your strength. Reflect on a recent moment when you were able to view your pain through a lens of safety. Describe the emotions and thoughts you experienced. Identify the specific tools that supported you.

_____

_____

_____

_____

Validate your experience. What thoughts or doubts typically arise during challenging episodes? How would you validate a friend going through a similar experience?

_____

_____

_____

_____

Empower yourself. Identify positive qualities within yourself. How can these qualities help you navigate future challenges?

_____

_____

_____

_____

Reassure and create safety. What self-assuring phrases resonate from your self-talk minis? Craft a reassuring message to yourself emphasizing safety.

_____

_____

_____

_____

Now write your empowering letter. Begin with a personal greeting. Reflect on the insights you gained from the previous prompts. Then write to yourself using your soothing self-talk tone, with validation, empowerment, reassurance, and safety. Incorporate self-assuring phrases like the self-talk minis you've identified. Conclude with a reminder of your strength and with encouragement to keep going.

Keep this letter on hand as a personal source of comfort and strength during tough moments, and return to it whenever you're in need of a confidence boost.

Extinction bursts, though challenging, signal your nervous system recalibrating for a breakthrough. Rather than see them as setbacks, you can recognize them as opportunities for mindful reframing, kindness, and deeper attunement to your internal experience. Recognize them as the indicators of progress that they are, like necessary turbulence before a smoother flight. In pain recovery, extinction bursts are old patterns resisting change, and each one is an opportunity to deepen your exploration and growth. Rewiring your brain is a challenging, nonlinear process, and understanding the ups and downs for what they are is the key to progress.

Navigating Recovery with Patience and Trust

Always remember that recovery and happiness are not about holding on tightly but about easing your grip. It's about allowing things to ebb and flow, with the understanding that the sought-after goal will, in its own time, find its way to you so long as you continue to walk the path.

Our belief in you is deep. Somewhere along our own journeys, someone expressed their belief in us (thank you, Alan). It's true you must believe in yourself. But if and when that belief wavers along the way, let our faith in your capacity to do this work buoy you—return to this workbook whenever you need it to light the way while you find your footing. And know that eventually, you will need to be your own light, and so long as you keep going, you definitely will be.

Acknowledgments

With heartfelt appreciation, we present this collaborative workbook, crafted by two women united in a common goal, bridging the gap of thousands of miles. Our shared commitment to doing what we can to change the way chronic pain is understood and treated, ignited by a passion for healing, permeates these pages, reflecting our common dedication to this work.

Our utmost admiration extends to esteemed mentors pivotal in shaping our work and this workbook: Alan Gordon, LCSW, creator of PRT and founder of the Pain Psychology Center; Drs. Donald Teater, Howard Schubiner, and David Clarke; PRT codeveloper Christie Uipi, LCSW; hypnotherapist Melany Cohen, LMFT; and Claudette Thor, LPC. Your combined expertise enriched every page as well as our professional journeys, and we extend gratitude for your invaluable contributions that guided us here.

Sincere respect and appreciation are offered to Drs. Yoni Ashar and Tor Wager and all other contributors to the Boulder Back Pain Study. Your research findings and insights have significantly enriched the field of chronic pain treatment, and we are so grateful.

To our exceptional team—graphic designer and friend, Joshua Wells, whose beautiful images infused the book with love, and our editors at New Harbinger, Ryan Buresh, Vicraj Gill, and Brady Kahn—thank you for bringing visual elegance and editorial finesse to this workbook.

A heartfelt acknowledgment goes to our unwavering support systems throughout the workbook's development. To Olivia's parents, Lois and Bob, her brother John, and husband, Kiel, for their bottomless love and support. To Vanessa's grandparents, Mark, Angie, Barbara, Harvey, and Myrna; sister Brianna; and partner Josh—you are my pillars of strength. To Elisa, Rob, and Nicole, Vanessa's chosen family, for your unconditional love.

Each of you played a vital role, and your patience and encouragement fueled the completion of this project.

With heartfelt gratitude, we thank our remarkable clients who have entrusted us with their healing. Whether currently in treatment, celebrating recovery, or facing challenges, your openness, trust, and resilience have been the driving force inspiring this endeavor. We do this for and because of you.

A special expression of gratitude goes to the exceptional therapists at the Pain Psychology Center, whose unwavering dedication to their clients' healing process motivates us to be creative, patient, and compassionate. Giovanna, Sherry, and John, thank you for everything you've done to encourage every bit of this process. And a special thank you to the brilliant members of the consultation group that originally brought us together.

And to our readers. We are truly grateful for this shared journey.

Additional Resources

Pain Psychology Center (PPC). The Pain Psychology Center specializes in pain recovery through a multidisciplinary approach, the only treatment center in the world that specializes in PRT for individualized, one-on-one support from a skilled psychotherapist or pain recovery coach. This workbook features inspiring stories from PPC clients, highlighting their journey toward pain recovery. Whether you are a provider or a prospective client, please follow this link to be connected: www.painpsychologycenter.com

Pain Reprocessing Therapy Center. Dedicated to training professionals from various disciplines in PRT, this center's aim is to empower providers globally with alternative tools beyond conventional models, enabling them to better assist their patients and clients. See their website for a worldwide directory of PRT practitioners: www.painreprocessingtherapy.com

Psychophysiologic Disorders Association (PPDA). Dr. David Clarke leads the PPDA, globally educating health professionals on evidence-based alternatives for chronic pain, functional syndromes, and unexplained symptoms. By focusing on stress, trauma, and emotions, the PPDA offers safer, more affordable, and effective solutions, contributing to ending the chronic pain epidemic and opioid crisis. Visit the PPDA website for a directory of health care providers trained in diagnosing and treating psychophysiologic disorders: www.ppdassociation.org

Dr. Howard Schubiner's Mind Body Medicine. Dr. Howard Schubiner, cocreator with Mark Lumley of Emotional Awareness and Expression Therapy (EAET), provides resources for recovery from pain-related conditions. Discover practical tools and insights to facilitate recovery by addressing emotional awareness and expression in the context of pain recovery: www.unlearnyourpain.com

Recovery Stories

Pain Brain. Documentary film following Alan Gordon, the developer of PRT, collaborating with neuroscientists to prove the effectiveness of this technique. Watch at: www.painbrainfilm.com

This Might Hurt. Documentary film following patients participating in Dr. Howard Schubiner's brain-based approach to healing chronic pain. Watch at: www.thismighthurtfilm.com

Like Mind, Like Body. Powered by Curable, this podcast is hosted by PRT codeveloper and founder of the Better Mind Center, Christie Uipi, LCSW, who interviews individuals, physicians, and researchers sharing powerful stories about the mind–body connection. Listen at: www.curablehealth.com/podcast

Tell Me About Your Pain Community. This Facebook group is a supportive space for individuals using PRT for chronic pain healing. Members share success stories, challenges, and receive skillful responses from those who have recovered. Join at: www.facebook.com/groups/695823314550483

Other Free Resources

The TMS Wiki 21-Day Pain Recovery Program by Alan Gordon, LCSW. This daily recovery program aims to help individuals reduce physical symptoms by demonstrating practical applications of theories. Access the program at: www.tmswiki.org/forum/painrecovery

The Steady Coach with Dr. Yonit Arthur, AuD. This resource empowers individuals with chronic dizziness through the free Healing Chronic Dizziness course and YouTube channel. You can also find more personalized support through group coaching, small group sessions, and one-on-one consultations. Explore resources at: www.thesteadycoach.com

Positively COVID with Amy Engkjer. The site offers a wealth of hopeful stories, mental health resources, and guidance for COVID recovery. Discover practical advice on rest, nutrition, movement, and maintaining hope in the face of challenges. Explore resources at: www.positivelycovid.org

References

Ashar, Y. K., A. Gordon, H. Schubiner, C. Uipi, K. Knight, Z. Anderson, J. Carlisle, et al. 2022. "Effect of Pain Reprocessing Therapy vs. Placebo and Usual Care for Patients with Chronic Back Pain: A Randomized Clinical Trial." *JAMA Psychiatry* 79(1): 13–23.

Bayer, T. L., P. E. Baer, and C. Early. 1991. "Situational and Psychophysiological Factors in Psychologically Induced Pain." *Pain* 44(1): 45–50.

Brinjikji, W., P. H. Luetmer, B. Comstock, B. W. Bresnahan, L. E. Chen, R. A. Deyo, S. Halabi, et al. 2015. "Systematic Literature Review of Imaging Features of Spinal Degeneration in Asymptomatic Populations." *American Journal of Neuroradiology* 36(4): 811–16.

Castro, W. H., S. J. Meyer, M. E. Becke, C. G. Nentwig, M. F. Hein, B. I. Ercan, S. Thomann, U. Wessels, and A. E. Du Chesne. 2001. "No Stress—No Whiplash? Prevalence Of "Whiplash" Symptoms Following Exposure to a Placebo Rear-End Collision." *International Journal of Legal Medicine* 114(6): 316–22.

Fisher, J. P., D. T. Hassan, and N. O'Connor. 1995. "Minerva." *BMJ* 310: 70.

Gordon, A., and A. Ziv. 2021. *The Way Out: A Revolutionary, Scientifically Proven Approach to Healing Chronic Pain.* New York: Avery.

Hashmi, J. A., M. N. Baliki, L. Huang, A. T. Baria, S. Torbey, K. M. Hermann, T. J. Schnitzer, and A. V. Apkarian. 2013. "Shape Shifting Pain: Chronification of Back Pain Shifts Brain Representation from Nociceptive to Emotional Circuits." *Brain* 136(9): 2751–68.

Raffaeli, W., and E. Arnaudo. 2017. "Pain as a Disease: An Overview." *Journal of Pain Research* 10: 2003–2008.

Schubiner, H., and M. Betzold. 2022. *Unlearn Your Pain: A 28-Day Process to Reprogram Your Brain*, 4th ed. Pleasant Ridge, MI: MindBody Publishing.

Schwartz, R. C. 2021. *No Bad Parts: Healing Trauma and Restoring Wholeness with the Internal Family Systems Model*. Louisville, CO: Sounds True.

———. 2023. *Introduction to Internal Family Systems,* 2nd ed. Louisville, CO: Sounds True.

Schwartz, R., R. Siegel, and H. Schubiner. 2021. "IFS and Chronic Pain: Listening to Inner Parts That Hold the Hurt." *Psychotherapy Networker*, January/February. https://www.psychotherapynetworker.org/article/ifs-and-chronic-pain.

Steffens, D., M. J. Hancock, C. G. Maher, C. Williams, T. S. Jensen, and J. Latimer. 2014. "Does Magnetic Resonance Imaging Predict Future Low Back Pain? A Systematic Review." *European Journal of Pain* 18(6): 755–65.

Vanessa M. Blackstone, MSW, citizen of the Eastern Band of Cherokee Indians Nation, is executive director of the Pain Psychology Center. She earned her MS in social work from the University of Southern California. Following her own personal recovery from chronic pain, Vanessa began her career as a therapist in 2018. She was one of the first clinical consultants at the Pain Reprocessing Therapy Center, and has helped train hundreds of practitioners in pain reprocessing therapy (PRT). In addition to chronic pain treatment, she specializes in sex therapy, substance use and recovery, mindfulness-based relapse prevention, and works on film sets as an on-set wellness professional. Outside of her professional roles, Vanessa is a former foster youth who advocates for current and former foster youth by sharing her personal experiences in public speaking events. She lives in Los Angeles, CA.

Olivia S. Sinaiko, LPC, leads the behavioral health pain program at the tribal health organization, Southeast Alaska Regional Health Consortium (SEARHC). She has been a featured presenter in the American Society of Addiction Medicine's (ASAM) training modules on nonpharmacological approaches to pain treatment and interdisciplinary care in the treatment of chronic pain, and has presented to the Pain Psychology Center on the relationship between attachment trauma and chronic pain. She earned her BA from Stanford University and her MA in counseling psychology from The Wright Institute, as well as a JD from Yale Law School. She lives in Juneau, AK.

Foreword writer **Alan Gordon, LCSW**, is a psychotherapist in Los Angeles, CA, specializing in the treatment of chronic pain and other physical symptoms. He is the developer of PRT, a cutting-edge protocol for treating chronic pain, and author of *The Way Out*. Gordon is also director of the Pain Psychology Center in Beverly Hills, CA; is an adjunct assistant professor at USC; and has presented on the topic of pain treatment at conferences and trainings throughout the country.

Real change *is* possible

For more than fifty years, New Harbinger has published proven-effective self-help books and pioneering workbooks to help readers of all ages and backgrounds improve mental health and well-being, and achieve lasting personal growth. In addition, our spirituality books offer profound guidance for deepening awareness and cultivating healing, self-discovery, and fulfillment.

Founded by psychologist Matthew McKay and Patrick Fanning, New Harbinger is proud to be an independent, employee-owned company. Our books reflect our core values of integrity, innovation, commitment, sustainability, compassion, and trust. Written by leaders in the field and recommended by therapists worldwide, New Harbinger books are practical, accessible, and provide real tools for real change.

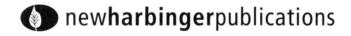 **newharbinger**publications

MORE BOOKS from
NEW HARBINGER PUBLICATIONS

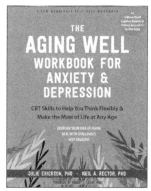

THE AGING WELL
WORKBOOK FOR ANXIETY
AND DEPRESSION

CBT Skills to Help You
Think Flexibly and Make the
Most of Life at Any Age

978-1648481260 / US $25.95

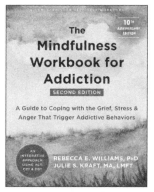

THE MINDFULNESS
WORKBOOK FOR ADDICTION,
SECOND EDITION

A Guide to Coping with
the Grief, Stress, and Anger That
Trigger Addictive Behaviors

978-1684038107 / US $24.95

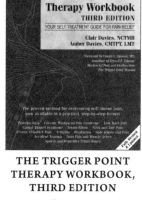

THE TRIGGER POINT
THERAPY WORKBOOK,
THIRD EDITION

Your Self-Treatment Guide
for Pain Relief

978-1608824946 / US $29.95

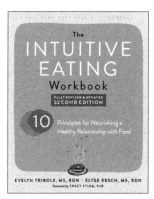

THE INTUITIVE
EATING WORKBOOK,
SECOND EDITION

Ten Principles for Nourishing a
Healthy Relationship with Food

978-1648484599 / US $26.95

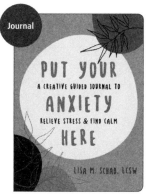

PUT YOUR
ANXIETY HERE

A Creative Guided Journal to
Relieve Stress and Find Calm

978-1648481451 / US $18.95

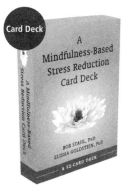

A MINDFULNESS-BASED
STRESS REDUCTION
CARD DECK

978-1684037797 / US $19.95

🌱 new**harbinger**publications

1-800-748-6273 / newharbinger.com

(VISA, MC, AMEX / prices subject to change without notice)
Follow Us 📷 👍 ✖ ▶ 📌 in ♪ ⑥

Don't miss out on new books from New Harbinger.
Subscribe to our email list at **newharbinger.com/subscribe** 👆

Did you know there are **free tools** you can download for this book?

Free tools are things like **worksheets**, **guided meditation exercises**, and **more** that will help you get the most out of your book.

You can download free tools for this book— whether you bought or borrowed it, in any format, from any source—from the New Harbinger website. All you need is a NewHarbinger.com account. Just use the URL provided in this book to view the free tools that are available for it. Then, click on the "download" button for the free tool you want, and follow the prompts that appear to log in to your NewHarbinger.com account and download the material.

You can also save the free tools for this book to your **Free Tools Library** so you can access them again anytime, just by logging in to your account! Just look for this button on the book's free tools page.

+ Save this to my free tools library